The Secrets of

Spiritual Marketing

*A Complete Guide for Natural
Therapists to Making Money Doing
What they Love*

T0204292

First published by O Books, 2009
O Books is an imprint of John Hunt Publishing Ltd., The Bothy, Deershot Lodge, Park Lane, Ropley,
Hants, SO24 0BE, UK
office1@o-books.net
www.o-books.net

Distribution in:

UK and Europe
Orca Book Services
orders@orcabookservices.co.uk
Tel: 01202 665432 Fax: 01202 666219
Int. code (44)

USA and Canada
NBN
custserv@nbnbooks.com
Tel: 1 800 462 6420 Fax: 1 800 338 4550

Australia and New Zealand
Brumby Books
sales@brumbybooks.com.au
Tel: 61 3 9761 5535 Fax: 61 3 9761 7095

Far East (offices in Singapore, Thailand,
Hong Kong, Taiwan)
Pansing Distribution Pte Ltd
kemal@pansing.com
Tel: 65 6319 9939 Fax: 65 6462 5761

South Africa
Stephan Phillips (pty) Ltd
Email: orders@stephanphillips.com
Tel: 27 21 4489839 Telefax: 27 21 4479879

Text copyright Lawrence Ellyard 2008

Design: Stuart Davies

ISBN: 978 1 84694 224 2

A CIP catalogue record for this book is available
from the British Library.

Printed by Digital Book Print

The Secrets of

Spiritual
Marketing

*A Complete Guide for Natural
Therapists to Making Money Doing
What they Love*

Lawrence Ellyard

Founder of the International Institute for
Complementary Therapists

BOOKS

Winchester, UK
Washington, USA

CONTENTS

Chapter 5

Chapter 6

About the author

Lawrence Ellyard is the CEO and Founder of the *International Institute for Complementary Therapists*. With over 15 years working as a natural therapy practitioner, instructor and educator, Lawrence combines this experience with his former background in Graphic Design, Advertising and Marketing.

The Secrets of Spiritual Marketing is his seventh book.

Visit: www.lawrenceellyard.com

Disclaimer

The material in this publication is of a general nature. It neither purports nor intends to be advice. Readers should not act on the basis of any matter in this publication without advice from either a licensed financial planner or a marketing professional, with due regard to their own particular circumstances. The author and publisher expressly disclaim all and any liability to any person, whether a purchaser of this publication or not, in respect of anything and of the consequence of anything done or omitted to be done by any such person in reliance, whether whole or partial, upon the whole or any part of the contents of this publication.

Dedication

This book is dedicated to all those talented therapists and practitioners who are great at doing what they do. May this book help you to share your gifts with many people so the benefit grows far and wide.

Praise for the Secrets of Spiritual Marketing

Lawrence Ellyard has created a fantastic business and marketing guide which marries proven marketing techniques with one's spiritual path. Without needing to compromise on your values, The Secrets of Spiritual Marketing will drive your wellness business through the roof.
- **Marci Shimoff**, NY Times bestselling author of Happy for No Reason and featured teacher in the hit movie The Secret

Lawrence Ellyard's newest book is a wonderfully down-to-earth, practical and user friendly tool-box for establishing, growing and flour-ishing a natural health business in integrity and truth. This book is a real gift to practitioners in all fields of healing.
- **Brandon Bays**, Author of The Journey and Freedom Is

The Secrets of Spiritual Marketing is a must for anyone working in the wellness industry. Full of useful tips for natural therapists or anyone in small business. This book lays the foundations for success.
- **Gary Quinn**, Author of Living in the Spiritual Zone.

This book's a gem! If you are serious about succeeding in business as a natural therapist, whether you are just starting out or established and looking to expand, you will find The Secrets of Spiritual Marketing by industry insider Lawrence Ellyard, of great value. This book offers sound marketing advice that will help you guide clients to your door, build and maintain a reputation for excellent customer service, and attract spiritual prosperity.
Thank you, Lawrence Ellyard!
- **Amy Z. Rowland**, Usui Reiki Master and author of Reiki for the Heart and Soul.

The Secrets of Spiritual marketing is a must-read for any natural therapist who is planning and running their own business, with the aim of improving the bottom line and achieving fulfillment.
- **Pamela Allardice**, Editor of Nature and Health Magazine.

Fantastic secrets to know before you start, I wish I had known. Straight forward and efficient. This book will save you hours and hours.
- **Diane Riley**, co-founder of the Australian School of Tantra and Author of Sexy and Sacred.

The Secrets of Spiritual Marketing is a book designed to help natural therapists to expand their practices and reach more people. Highly recommended!
- **David Vennells**, Author of The Healing Sourcebook.

Lawrence Ellyard has done what for many has proven to be one of the most difficult areas in their lives - marrying their spiritual/holistic work with the world of business and marketing. This in depth, step-by-step guide to setting up and running a prosperous wellness business is both timely and required reading for anyone in the health and healing industry.
- **Leo Drioli**, Editor of Innerself Newspaper

There is nothing more difficult then starting your own practice without marketing guidance like this. I believe The Secrets of Spiritual Marketing is a must read for every natural therapist wanting to create a successful practice!
- **Adria Ellis**, Founder of Zen Alliance Natural Health Directory.

Covers something truly unique. A must read for every natural therapist.
- **Mette Sorensen**, Founder of Mette's Institute for Ka Huna Massage.

A must-read for all natural therapists either starting their own practice or those already established. Industry expert Lawrence Ellyard shares his secrets on how to gain and maintain business success and prosperity in the wellness industry, whilst maintaining your spiritual integrity. Time-saving, tried and tested tools that will see your business soar! I highly recommend it.
- **Suzanne Taylor**, Publisher of the Natural Health Directory Australia.

Lawrence's latest book, Spiritual Marketing, is constructive, earthed, practical and is an extremely comprehensive resource for any new health practitioner. It's going to be a book that will remain on your practice bookshelf, dog-eared and laden with annotations for many years as your practice grows and flourishes utilising Lawrence's obvious wisdom.
- **Ian Hamilton**, Director of ION LIFE.

Any practitioner, new graduate or seasoned natural therapist can learn from the valuable information clearly provided in The Secrets of Spiritual Marketing. The website chapter is great for everyone in the natural health field. This industry needs the most professional face possible - good websites and marketing materials are essential for thera- pists and this guide is an excellent resource.
- **Bianca Rothschild**, Publisher of The Natural Health Guide Australia.

The Secrets of Spiritual Marketing is a comprehensive and user friendly compendium about building a successful and lucrative practice – the easy way. These fantastic marketing ideas and hands on advice will help any Natural Therapist to build their business and client base in the most cost effective way and ensure a smooth transition from being student to becoming a professional health care provider. This book is a must for anyone who is serious about doing what they love for a living.
- **Katha Jones**, Director of International Institute of Kinesiology Australia.

The Secrets of Spiritual Marketing is a book that will be most beneficial to natural therapists already in business as well as new therapists alike. I wish I had access to something as easy and informative to follow when I was starting out in my practice.
- **Keitha Bradley**, Founder of Open Gate Natural Therapy School Australia.

Heaps of practical and useful advice for the beginning as well as seasoned practitioner. Lawrence Ellyard's secrets applied will direct any natural therapy business towards soaring success. Recommended reading for our students.
- **Ki'a'i Ho'okahi Weber**, Founder of Australian College of Kahuna Sciences.

A timely and powerful body of work by Lawrence Ellyard. In 'The Secrets of Spiritual Marketing' Lawrence shares his insights and wisdom to support the modern day wellness practitioner. His insights and honest sharing makes this book a must read for anyone in this industry.
- **Chris Hooper**, Founder of Chris Hooper Promotions and Management Australia.

Introduction

The Secrets of Spiritual Marketing is written for the talented and gifted natural therapists of this world. Truth be told, most natural therapists are excellent at what they do. They have undertaken all of the training in their chosen field, have spent hours in clinical practice and in many respects they are experts in facilitating their natural health therapy. However not all is well for the wellness professionals. When it comes to promoting and advertising their natural health therapy practice, most therapists are less than capable of effectively promoting and marketing what they do.

One of the primary reasons why natural therapists lack the ability to effectively promote themselves is simply due to the fact that little or no time is devoted to learning about marketing or advertising. It makes sense then that in order to successfully build a practice where we not only bring in new customers and clients but retain our existing clientele that we need to receive an education in achieving this.

Marketing by definition is the art of selling and is defined as being the business of delivering the goods (your services) from you (the producer) to the consumer.

Spiritual marketing is defined as a way to share what you love to do and be financially supported by providing your services in order to help others.

Because most natural therapists are poorly educated about advertising and promoting their natural therapy practice, they often look to what everyone else is doing. The result is more advertisements that fail to be effective simply because almost everyone is copying everyone else's badly written and poorly designed ads. The good news is, there is help. What you behold is a complete guide to effectively marketing your natural health therapy practice which will bring you lasting results and more clients than you could ever need.

Spiritual Marketing enables you to help people and to solve their problems through your experience and training. However, in order for you to help more people, they need to know that you exist. Spiritual Marketing provides you with methods to bring your wellness business to more people and thereby help others to live happy, healthy and more fulfilled lives.

If you can touch one person's life they will treat those around them in positive ways, and like a stone dropped into a still body of water, the ripples of your practice can touch more peoples' lives and you can be duly compensated for your talents. Isn't this our goal, to help others?

In preparation for writing this book, I interviewed many natural health therapists and asked them the question, *"Why do you do what you do?"* most people invariably answered that their main reason was to benefit others.

The thing is it is quite okay to be financially rewarded whilst helping others, it is actually a very spiritual thing – money, that is. Having issues with money is more common than most people think. We often think about our lack of funds before looking at other peoples' lack of financial abundance. This comes from the way many of us had the words drummed into our heads: *"You cannot be spiritual and wealthy"* or *"Money is the root of all evil"*.

I also hear from many therapists and healers that they do not charge for treatments because *"Money gets in the way of spirit"*. If a therapist chooses not to charge for their time then this is fine provided they have an alternative source of income. Some people prefer to have a natural therapy practice as a hobby and do so because they feel uncomfortable charging for their services, but let us take a look for a moment at the truth of Spiritual Marketing.

No matter what you do, whether you give counseling consultations or collect the garbage from the street, every profession involves helping others' solve their problems or offers a service to improve others lives. What most therapists don't realise is that all work, no matter what it is, is spiritual because it offers a solution to people's problems.

It does not matter what we do, we are all in some way in the business of helping others.

When it comes to practitioners in the natural therapy industry where we often find this mistaken view about money that somehow it is not spiritual (especially when it comes to a lot of money). It is important to recognise that whatever you do is by definition is a spiritual practice. I should point out that a lot of the people who have issues with charging for their services are usually the ones who have lack in their financial abundance. In some cases they use the excuse of being spiritual to perpetuate the continued lack of financial success.

Over the years I have also heard from many people in the wellness industry as well as from many other spiritual and new age arts that they do not consider it spiritual to earn from their spiritual practice, let alone make a lot of money from their practice. They feel that receiving money by giving treatments is directly violating spiritual laws.

What many fail to see is that abundance is our birthright and being abundant *is* spiritual. One need only look at nature to see the wealth so clearly displayed. When a flower blooms it does not hold back and only reveal a few petals, it opens fully and reveals itself completely. It really is our birthright to be abundant and that also means that prosperity is simply a manifestation of this abundance. We should use this wealth wisely and ensure we use this money in ways to benefit both ourselves and our community.

Money is a symbol of value and an exchange of energy, and nothing more. Money gives you choices and options. It is very hard to help the poor and needy by being poor and needy ourselves. By the same token when you find another person stuck down a well, you will be of little help by jumping in with them. Being financially wealthy is like having a ladder to help rescue the person who is in the well and calling for help.

When we look at what holds people back from being financially successful in their natural therapy practice, we find the biggest thing standing in their way are self-limiting beliefs around prosperity. It is a well known spiritual law that *'as we think, so we become'* and this especially applies to our self-worth regarding our financial abundance and prosperity.

If you are going to succeed in your natural therapy practice, not only spiritually but financially, then you need to alter your mindset from one of lack, to one of adbundance. It is important to recognise that in order for you to share your spiritual gifts with as many people as you can and thereby help them, then it is logical that those people first need to be able to reach you. This is exactly what Spiritual Marketing is.

You can get started on becoming successful by looking at your beliefs around money.

The simple logic is to ask yourself: *'Why do I wish to begin a natural therapy practice?'*

When we ask ourselves this question some of our answers might include:

'To help others who are in need'
'To grow in myself by healing others'
'To be a spiritual example to others'
'To improve my abilities by working with other people'

Your reasons may include these or you may have other reasons. Whatever the reasons are, promoting yourself is inevitable if you are going to benefit others.

Your services also need to be reciprocal. It is important to closely examine the benefit of exchange. When you offer a service to another, you set in motion a benefit to that person's life. As a result they will be more able to benefit others. The fact that you have helped them means that they, in accordance with the law of *karma* (or cause and effect) owe you something in return. When we charge for our services we create an opportunity for the recipient to return our gift and thus create a karmic balance. It is actually your responsibility to charge for your services, thereby creating perfect balance and an equal exchange for services rendered.

Most people in the natural therapy industry focus a great deal of time and energy on cultivating their skills in of their chosen field. But the fact is that it doesn't matter how good you are at what you do if nobody knows about it.

What I have also encountered amongst many natural therapists who work in the wellness industry is that most do not earn enough or do not have enough clients to earn the kind of lifestyle they desire. Some have a complacent attitude to their financial situation, thinking that in order to do what you love to do they cannot become wealthy doing it. I am here to tell you that this is simply not true.

By applying the tried and tested techniques presented in this book you can 'have your cake and eat it too'. I have seen too many excellent practitioners go out of business simply because they lacked both the belief and the methodology to bring their wellness business out of poverty into prosperity. The only thing that prevents you is the will and the proven tools presented in *The Secrets of Spiritual Marketing*.

The wellness industry is today one of the fastest growing industries. There is a new trend towards complementary therapies where the emphasis is on prevention of illness and support of our health, rather than just a last minute cure. With the growing trend towards preventative medicine particularly in the natural health industry, people are looking for something more which is not only about enhancing their lifestyle, but taking preventive action to enhance and maintain health in order to live a more balanced and healthier life.

The opportunities for natural health practitioners to make a living in the wellness industry are better today than ever before and conversely there are many more wellness industry practitioners in practice. This presents a great variety of natural therapy options in the market place for consumers, which also equals greater competition for natural therapists. How will you make your business stand out from the crowd?

This book highlights some of the well guarded marketing secrets. Some of the concepts provided in this book fly in the face of traditional marketing techniques yet are tried and tested techniques which work and continue to work to bring you new clients who retain their loyalty.

When it comes to finding new clients some statistics report that it is ten times harder to obtain a new client than it is to get a repeat purchase from an existing client for your product or service. With this in mind, we can do many things to retain our existing clientele and entice them in many exciting ways to purchase again and again. The techniques offered in this book illustrate the importance of providing an excellent service and also suggest a variety of compelling benefits which your customers will find hard to resist. By utilising the suggestions in this book your profits will increase, plus your customers will happily pay for your services.

The methods presented in this book have been used in business just like yours with great success for many years. The techniques I share have also worked for me. Having been in practice as a natural therapist and educator of natural therapies for over 15 years, I have successfully utilised these techniques over and over with enormously positive results. This has not only translated to an increase in clients but a definite increase in tangible profits as well.

Of course, with any of the strategies presented in this book you have to see if it fits your business and with what you are trying to achieve. This is why I always recommend three things when trying any of these techniques. These are: Test, Test and Test. We need to test and re-test the marketing techniques we use to ensure we are getting the most value from our advertising and marketing approaches.

The following chapters are in many respects stand alone topics so if you know that what you really need to do to improve your business is focus on building your website, or you sense that the vital improvement will be from looking after your existing clients, then you need not read through the book from cover to cover. Simply use your time to the most benefit and skip ahead to the chapters which are relevant to your business right now.

Over the years I have spent thousands of dollars in research and training in the pursuit of these highly prized and guarded secrets which you now hold in your hands. I believe these secrets should be made available to everyone in our industry. So this is my gift to you. Your end of the bargain is to put these sound ideas into action!

I wish you well with your spiritual and business life for the two go hand in hand.

Lawrence Ellyard
Fremantle, Western Australia
February 2009

Chapter 1

Establishing your Professional Practice

Before we embark upon our journey into the Secrets of Spiritual Marketing we first need to establish some foundations about a professional natural therapy practice. This first chapter will give you some insights into establishing a professional practice as well as covering a variety of options you may or may not have considered.

Are you ready to establish a professional practice?

At some point you will need to make a decision as to whether you prefer to practice your therapy as a hobby among your family and friends, or are a professional practitioner. Many natural therapists often begin as a hobby practitioner giving sessions in their spare time, only to find that they become increasingly popular and naturally move from hobby to professional out of demand. Other practitioners go into their training in natural therapies as a vocation with the sole reason to make it their livelihood and career.

As such, establishing a professional practice is something which either evolves or is decided upon from the outset. It goes without saying that one should attain a certain degree of experience and training prior to taking this important step. For practitioners who intend to establish a professional practice, it is recommended to wait until they have completed their training and have the necessary experience when giving treatments to join the professional body and take out professional insurances, before offering one's services to the general public for a fee.

In order to give treatments in a professional manner, one requires a treatment room in which to practice. It is necessary to

9

create a special space for your therapy practice in order to convey a professional and experienced approach and one that will support the healing for others. There are many options, which I will touch on later in this chapter.

How do I get started?

To set up your business you will need to decide whether you wish to be a sole trader or to form a company from which to trade under. It is recommended that you first contact your accountant for advice on whether you should be a sole trader or form a company structure. In addition, these are some other important considerations:

- You will need to decide whether to work under the banner of a health center, whether to open your own clinic and private practice, or be a mobile therapist, or an on-site therapist.
- In order to practice you will need a venue, whether this is from your home or rented rooms.
- You will need promotional materials such as business cards as well as the necessary practitioner equipment according to your modality.
- You will need to register your business with the tax office and register a business name to trade your business under.
- Once you have registered your business name you will also need to establish a bank account. Then you will need to make decisions on what kind of account you wish to have and how you will receive money for your services. This includes whether you require merchant facilities where you can receive credit card payments and whether you will choose to have a cheque book or receive payments only in cash.
- You will need to decide whether you want a secure post office box for receiving mail which ensures better privacy

for you as a personal individual beyond your practice, or whether you wish to receive correspondence to your residential address or work address. Or you may wish only to receive correspondence via email. In most cases you'll also need an email address dedicated to your practice which is preferably linked to your newly created website.

- You will need to make a decision on how people will reach you via the telephone, whether you'll offer a toll free 1800 number, or whether will have a landline (with answer phone to leave messages or a receptionist to take bookings) or whether you wish to only receive enquiries via a designated cell phone.

- You will need to determine what kind of advertising and marketing you wish to take out, and what your budget for this will be weekly, monthly, and annually.

- You will need to determine what your out-going expenses will be and what start up costs you will need in order to get your business up and running.

Put simply, there is so much to consider when establishing a new business but this is not the aim of this book. There are so many excellent books on the market about starting a small business. A good place to start is the 'Dummies' series such as *Small Business for Dummies*. You will also find some additional books in the recommended reading section at the end of this book to help get you started.

Joining associations and gaining professional affiliations

In addition to regular practise and upgrading your training in natural therapies, it is also advisable to be affiliated with organisations, associations and institutes related to your field of study. The colleges which offer professional training are a starting place for this information and of course the internet is a wonderful resource when it comes to finding associations. Simply type *'Natural Therapy Associations'* in a search engine such as: www.google.com and you will find a number from which to choose.

By joining an association that represents your chosen modalities in the natural health industry you gain valuable credibility and a professional affiliation.

The benefits of joining associations for natural therapies include:

- The ability to advertise your affiliation with the professional body.
- Access to health fund rebates for your clients who are covered through private health cover.
- Access to continued professional education and training.
- The ability to operate under the code of ethics of your association and aligning yourself with other recognised practitioners conveying a high standard of practice in natural therapies.
- As an affiliated practitioner you will have the right to take out practitioner indemnity insurance which is usually discounted through the association.

Depending upon the particular association or professional body* there are numerous other benefits but these are the standard ones practitioners can benefit from.

The International Institute for Complementary Therapists, of whom the author is the founder and director, offers membership and professional affiliation for over 550 natural therapy modalities throughout Australia and New Zealand. You can find out more information by visiting: www.iict.com.au

Practitioner insurance

If you are serious about your natural therapy practice then it is advisable (and in some countries it is mandatory) to have Practitioner Liability Insurance. Many associations now offer Practitioner Insurance as part of their membership benefits which enables you the benefits of professional affiliation and insurance for your practice.

Namely, one should obtain practitioner insurance which protects you for Public Liability and Professional Indemnity as well as Products Liability where applicable.

These terms are often misunderstood or seen as 'insurance jargon' so if you are wondering what these mean then the following is a brief explanation:

Public Liability means that whilst receiving a treatment (or whilst on your premises) a client injures themselves, for example by falling off your treatment table or tripping over the front steps on your property. In such an event you are covered if they sue you for damages.

Professional Indemnity covers all professional risk. This means that if for some reason, the person you are treating is injured as a direct result of your treatment, or claims this to be the case you are covered in the event of damages being awarded against you.

Product Liability covers you for any products you may use during your treatment, such as foot creams, massage oils or lotions, flower essences, pillows or steam cures.

If you are operating from premises such as a health centre, or from your home, it is worth considering insurance. Although many natural therapists would scoff at the very notion that their therapy could harm anyone, one needs to be aware that there are those unhappy people who might make such claims against your practice. Although the risk is considerably low, it is still worth insuring your business as you never know when litigation may rise up against you and cripple your finances, sometimes for life.

Besides insurance, it is also important to be conscious of any practical health and safety measures which may prevent accidents from occurring. If you operate from a premises, be sure to check the environment for any 'accidents waiting to happen'. For example, a loose carpet, an unsafe treatment table, slippery floors, or electrical power cords trailing in the path of people who may be walking through the room or high traffic areas like a staircase or landing. Keeping a safe workplace is a simple task of assessing your environment and making conscious changes where needed.

There are many insurance companies who now insure practitioners and teachers of natural therapies. When looking for practitioner insurance, be sure to get a number of quotes and to make sure the insurance company understands exactly what you are offering. You will find that prices vary from a few hundred dollars to thousands, so it is worth shopping around for the best quote to suit your practice needs.

Health fund rebates

In addition to joining an association you may also qualify for health fund rebates which your practice can offer as an added benefit for your clients. Providing health fund rebates will save your clients money on their treatments and is an excellent feature to ensure their loyalty to your practice. Today, more and more natural therapies are being recognised by private health funds and many offer considerable rebates to customers who use complementary therapies.

In order to obtain health provider status you need to be practicing a natural therapy modality which is recognised by the health funds and private health insurers in your country. Most practitioners belong to an association for natural therapies as a means to obtain automatic recognition for health fund provider status. Other practitioners apply on the merits of their qualifications without being represented under the banner of an association for recognition. The best way to determine whether you qualify for the health provider status is to contact your preferred natural therapy association to see if they offer members automatic recognition. Alternatively, contact the health funds in your country for more information.

Establishing your treatment room

Although a treatment room is not always requirement in order to give a treatment for natural therapies, a space dedicated to your practice can greatly increase not only the meditative qualities and relaxation of the treatment, but will also provide you with a professional edge for your practice in the eyes of the public.

If you choose to establish a treatment room, the following are some guidelines which you may find useful:

- Select a room away from busy areas.
- Create a safe, relaxing, and quiet space. Use soft colours, with light blinds over windows to create ambience.
- Plants can also help create a natural atmosphere.
- Depending upon the treatment you may also wish to use lighting for effect or light candles to help create a calm atmosphere.

In terms of practitioner equipment, you may require:

- A massage treatment table.
- A comfortable rolling chair (preferably height adjustable), if seated for giving your treatments.
- Pillows for added comfort and a light blanket if your client feels cool during the treatment.
- Sufficient towels when conducting massage treatments,

for example
- A box of tissues in case your client has a runny nose or feels emotional.
- A selection of soothing music *(be sure to have music which your client finds relaxing)*.
- Aromatherapy diffuser and oils to add pleasant aromas and aid in relaxation. Be sure to find out if your client has any allergies and always avoid cheap aromatherapy products.

Avoid:

- Pets entering your treatment space if you are conducting sessions from your home.
- Mobile phones (both yours and your clients) ringing during a treatment session; make it a habit to ensure that they are switched off or turned to silent during the treatment.
- Interruptions from family members and children if you are working from home, and from the receptionist or other colleagues if you are working from a centre or clinic. Place a sign on your door to indicate that a session is in progress and advise those around you so as to avoid unnecessary interruptions during the treatment.

Massage treatment tables
If your treatments make use of a massage treatment table then quality and functionality is essential. This is perhaps the most important piece of equipment that you will ever buy for your natural therapy practice and one that you should therefore not skimp on quality when buying it. By purchasing a sound treatment table, your table will feature some practical options for a professional practice. Your table should ideally feature a face hole or head cradle when your client needs to receive a treatment

face down. You may also consider a footstool to enable your client's easy access up on to the couch and down again after the treatment, and a height adjustable stool which will enable your easy access to your client when they are lying down.

The correct height for your treatment table will ensure you will be in a comfortable position when giving treatments for extended periods of time. Because many treatments involve positioning the hands on the body, many practitioners opt for a height adjustable stool as this is easier on the legs and especially the arms as you can use the table to lean your elbows on if giving treatments seated.

It is also worth mentioning that when giving treatments one should position the treatment table in the room so it is possible for you to move with ease all the way around it, enabling you full access to every position without unnecessarily disturbing your client.

Music

Another important part of a treatment experience may include the use of ambient music. If music features in your treatments, it is important to choose music that is fairly level throughout. The last thing you need is a track which is full of sudden surprises like increased tempo or rapid drumming. Although music with mantras or chanting can be of benefit as their repetitive nature will take both the giver and receiver into a deep and peaceful state of mind, in general music which does not have lyrics is best as you may find that both you and your client focus on the words, which can prevent deeper states of consciousness being reached.

Ask your client what types of music they find restful and remember to play their favourite music from your collection when giving on-going treatments, or encourage them to bring a CD of their own favourite music.

Where to practice

Establishing a practice can take many forms and there are several options ranging from your home, renting space at an established clinic, or practicing as a mobile therapist, to name a few.

This following section has been adapted from Steven Harold's book - Marketing Tips for Complementary Therapists, which is an excellent guide well worth reading. The next section provides an overview of some options for your consideration.

Your home

For practitioners on a budget, starting a practice from home has its advantages as one will not incur extra rental costs to hire a room. Your home is generally more comfortable and familiar to you and you need not travel in order to give a treatment.

Other benefits include:

- Greater flexibility in appointment times, as you can fit clients into your schedule.
- You do not have any long term contract agreements as is often the case when hiring a room in a healing centre or office.

Although there are benefits, practicing from home also has its downfalls.

These include:

- The potential disruptions from family (children), friends dropping in, life laundry such as meter readings and washing machine repair men, or pets disrupting your session or disturbing your client.
- You are inviting clients into your personal space – this may lead to a sense of invasion of privacy for you or other family members in your household.

- You will need to have the space to set aside a room in your home to be exclusively used for your treatments, or one which can be tidied of all signs of family life to be your therapy room.
- Your clients may question your professionalism as you may not be able to offer a waiting room or reception service if they arrive a few minutes early, or you over run a session.
- There are the potential problems from your local council, which may not allow you to run a business from home, as well as parking issues.
- You may be unlucky to have noisy neighbours or even worse, disgruntled neighbours.

Renting a room

When considering the option of renting a room, whether this is from a complementary therapy centre or office, there are again pros and cons.

Some of the advantages in renting a room include:

- You will not have the problem of potential interruptions from family members and you may have the option of having a receptionist who can take bookings for you all week leading up to the days when you are in the clinic (*this adds tremendous credibility to your practice*).
- There will be a waiting room if clients arrive early and you can often network your client base with other therapists in the same building and refer clients for treatment to other modalities if you feel this will be beneficial for their healing.
- Many centres also have the option of credit card facilities for easy payments by your clients.
- Someone else – the receptionist – will take the payments for you, which saves you time for working with your next

client and also saves the discomfort of taking money if you prefer not to be so closely associate with the business side of your practice.

- You can rent the room for the number of mornings / afternoons that your practice will be full, and thereby share the rent of your room with another practitioner, while also having your space set up for the sole purpose of treating others.

Of course, there are some disadvantages as well.

These include:

- The costs and commitments to paying for a room to practice from. You may not always get a constant flow of clients and will need to pay the rent regardless of whether it is a busy or quiet month.
- You may not have as much freedom to see your clients 'outside hours' as the room may only be available at certain times.
- You will have to travel to and from your practice.
- There is the potential problem of your practice being located on a busy street or highway thus adding to the problem of noise and parking issues.
- There may be 'office politics' in the practice as in any workplace, for example you may be dissatisfied with the receptionist's manner or efficiency, or there may be differing opinions between practitioners as to how the clinic should advertise.

Some other things to consider when choosing premises to practice from include:

- Client accessibility – is the location easy to get to from bus routes and train lines?

- Does your room have access to wheelchair and disability ramps and toilets?
- What is the parking like and is it close to your centre?
- Are there time limits for parking or parking problems which may be expensive and might discourage clients from booking to see you at that clinic?

You will also need to determine when most people will be able to see you for treatments; and whether you will only offer treatments during office hours or also during the evenings or on weekends. You will also need to determine whether your treatment room will be available during these preferred times.

The other thing to consider is the overall appearance of your treatment room. You can add much credibility to your practice if you make the room a sanctuary for relaxation and peace. You can do much to add peaceful ambience to your room. Use your creativity and ask other practitioners for feedback. A fresh pair of eyes and some honest feedback on your treatment room can be very rewarding.

Mobile therapist

Another way to practice is to become a mobile therapist. A mobile therapist means that you are available to travel to your clients to offer treatments in the comfort of their home or work place.

Mobile therapists can actually tap new clientele which may include:

- The elderly.
- Mothers with small children at home.
- People with disabilities.
- People who lack transport.
- People in hospitals or hospices.
- People in offices, businesses or workplaces such as

airports for a corporate clientele.

- People who have phobias such as the fear of open spaces (agoraphobia) or fears of public transport, such as riding on trains.

There are many advantages to being a mobile therapist. These include:

- No rental costs for hiring a room or a lease contract to tie you down.
- You will reach more people.
- Your clients will feel more comfortable being treated in the comfort of their own home or office.

Some of the disadvantages may include:

- You may not have all the facilities at hand that you require to provide your treatment comfortably.
- You will incur additional travel costs and spend time traveling to and from your client's home or office.
- You will be giving your treatment in an unfamiliar setting with no real idea of what arrangement you will encounter upon arrival. This will also take extra time to set up for the treatment session.
- You will need to transport your treatment table and other equipment everywhere you go.
- You might encounter the annoyance of turning up to give your session only to find your client is not at home or has forgotten about your appointment or even given you the wrong address!

When it comes to avoiding missed treatments a very effective way to counter this is to arrange payment prior to giving the treatment. This not only secures your costs, it is a sure way of guaranteeing that your client will be there when you show up. Many mobile therapists add an additional fee to cover travel expenses or add the time it takes to travel at their usual hourly rate.

In order to counter some of the potential problems with carting your practitioner equipment around you might encourage a regular client to purchase their own treatment table or treatment equipment. It might sound strange but you will be surprised how accommodating some people can be. I know a mobile Remedial Massage therapist who has several clients who supply their own treatment table in their homes. They do this because he is simply that good at what he does and they feel they are getting the very best treatment by having all the right equipment for it.

Working as an on-site therapist

Examples of on-site therapist settings include: staff treatments in large offices, mine sites, and corporate events. If you are fortunate enough to be offered a position as an on-site therapist, there are numerous benefits which include inheriting an already established client base. This means that you will have no marketing or advertising costs at the outset (although you will need to do some self-promoting to keep these contracts flowing in, and you may also choose to do some on-going promotional work to let people know where you are in demand).

The company will promote you, thus ensuring on-going work as well as the inevitable referrals which will come via 'word of mouth'. This can translate into obtaining further private treatments outside your on-site practice.

Chapter 2

How Much to Charge for your Services

Now that we have looked at the various options of how and where you can establish a natural therapy practice this following section explores the all important subject of charging for your services.

Many new natural therapy practitioners who take the step of charging for their services often have some difficulty determining a fair value for their treatments. Many sell themselves short by thinking that they are but an instrument for the universe and consider it un-spiritual to charge a reasonable fee for their services. However, the amount we charge should be indicative of our level of expertise, experience, and training.

One way to determine your worth is to call on others who are practicing the same natural therapy and ask them what they charge. By doing this you will also get an idea of what the accepted fee structure is for your location, level of expertise, and the fees that can reasonably be charged for your natural therapy modality.

It is also important to set the right fee. Setting a fee that is too low can actually backfire and as a result your clients may assume you are 'not as good' and so undervalue your service and the benefit of your therapy. They may also think that you do not have enough experience or lack credible training if your price is under-valued.

Setting a fee that is too high on the other hand, will 'price yourself out of the market' and leave potential clients being unable to afford your services. Therefore you must strike a suitable balance so that your clients will value your services and be able to afford them on a regular basis.

Once you have established your treatment fee, you may need

to review this from time to time to take into account increased costs, such as room rental. It is normal for businesses to increase their prices every second year, so the same should apply to your business.

Practitioner expenses

When you are determining your fee structure you also need to factor in all your expenses. These might include:

- Government taxes.
- Rent for your room and service charges.
- Travel expenses and fuel.
- Maintaining your practitioner equipment.
- Washing towels and treatment couch covers.
- Paying your practitioner insurances.
- Advertising costs.
- Business stationery.
- Printing and promotional materials.
- Postage.
- Telephone bills and mobile phone.
- Website and Internet access.

Concessions

Some practitioners like to offer concessions for seniors, students, and the unemployed. The decision to offer concessions is ultimately your decision. When you do offer a concession this means you receive less income per hour for your time. An alternative to offering discounts is to create special offers. Special offers can actually increase your hourly rate by creating additional business because your special offer will entice your clients to have a repeat treatment. When we add a value or incentive to what we offer we actually create more business for ourselves. Always follow the 'up-sell' option.

Some offers might include a VIP earnings card, where your

5th treatment is free. Other incentives may include a 10% discount when three treatments are paid in advance. Either way, special offers like this mean you will give more treatments which equals repeat business for you. We will explore a number of up-sell options and other ways to entice your clients to return to you time and again in chapter 11.

Rules of practice – Cancellations and confirmations

Once we have determined our financial worth we need to determine the rules for payment. One way to avoid missed treatments where your client cancels or simply forgets to come for the appointment is to phone, email or send a text message the day before to confirm the appointment time. It only takes a moment of your time and you can avoid any issues with missed appointments.

However it is inevitable that at some time during your practice your client will cancel an appointment and in some cases, just not show up. You need to determine whether you charge a cancellation fee. Many practitioners require 24 hours cancellation notice. In the event that a client calls more than 12 hours prior to their appointment some may opt for a 50% cancellation fee, whilst other practitioners choose to take the cancellation in their stride and waive any charge.

One way to counter the problem of cancellations or missed appointments is to secure payment prior to the appointment. Credit card bookings over the phone are a great way to achieve this. You can be sure that if your client has paid in advance, they will move mountains to get there and even if they don't, your time is paid for all the same.

Some practitioners may argue that they would never consider charging a cancellation fee, thinking that they will lose their client, however you need to consider your time and the preparation it takes to give a treatment.

Consider these points:

- You should be compensated when you have arranged your day around your clients booking.
- You should be compensated for lost appointments, when another client might otherwise have booked that session time.
- You should be compensated for the time it takes to set up your treatment room and for the mental preparation it takes to give a treatment.
- However you may decide that illness is unavoidable and your clients should not be penalised for being sick, and allow the appointment to be rescheduled for another day.

You will need to effectively communicate your cancellation policy over the phone when the booking is made, as well as having your payment terms and conditions clearly displayed in your treatment room or office, so reducing any potential misunderstandings.

Getting paid and payment options

It is often at the end of giving a treatment that most practitioners settle the account. However, you may wish to do this when your client arrives. For many people, there may be some tension about money. By sorting out the payment prior to the treatment or well in advance, money becomes one less thing to think about.

In my experience after receiving a treatment, your client may be in a vulnerable state or in a highly peaceful and relaxed state. On a number of occasions I have completely forgotten about the payment, not realizing until the client is long gone. Settling the account prior to your consultations solves such problems.

Another good reason for this is that you may not wish for your client to have to deal with money after the treatment. In this way, they can simply leave to enjoy the serene state of mind after the treatment.

Credit card payments

It is becoming more common to use credit card facilities to make payments and it seems this will only increase more so in the future. Therefore, it makes good business sense to have these facilities at your disposal. If you have many clients, electronic facilities save time and present a more professional image.

Besides, by far the easiest way to secure payments for your services is via credit card. This can be obtained over the phone, online via a secure payment gateway such as *paypal,* or in person.

Provided you have some financial history most banks will approve the use of merchant facilities for your business. With credit card facilities, you will be able to receive payments for your treatments over the phone, as well as mail order, or internet payments for advanced bookings.

If you cannot obtain credit card facilities you may wish to arrange payment via internet paypal or internet banking where your client pays for the treatment in advance into your nominated bank account. In order to achieve this you will need to advise your client of your banking details for deposits. One disadvantage to consider is that it often takes three business days for payments made to register on your account. This makes the payment well in advance the better rule of thumb.

If you take cheques, be sure to write their cheque guarantee card number on the back – even if they are a long standing client they may have a deficit in their bank account that month and a guaranteed cheque will ensure you are paid even if it is by overdraft. If it is a new client it is a good idea to ask the receptionist to put your client's address and contact details on the back of the cheque. This adds some security in cases where the cheque 'bounces'. You will be glad you requested this as you will have a record and a way of making contact with your client to ensure you actually get paid. Some business owners simply avoid this issue by not accepting payment via this method.

Online payment options

If you have a website (and you should) then it is ideal to establish an online shop for bookings. If you do your research on this you may find that prices vary considerably from highly unaffordable to slightly more affordable. It really becomes a question of whether you have enough monthly turn-over to warrant having an online payment facility.

The fact is that most people these days are making bookings online. Whether you choose to offer a simple booking form, where your clients can enter their credit card details via a secure server or a shopping cart system, both forms work considerably well.

Being a credit card society, more and more people are using credit cards in their day to day purchases. If you can go down to the local supermarket and buy your groceries with a credit card then why not use the same method to pay for your natural therapy treatments?

Cash

An increasingly rare method of payment but some clients simply prefer to pay for their treatments in cash. This of course is a wonderful thing. Although you may advertise that you offer credit card facilities you should not limit your business to only receiving payments in this way. Cash creates 'cash flow' which enables you direct access to funds that can be re-invested into your business and promotional activities. You can also use cash for your everyday expenses.

Of course, one should always play by the rules and declare your cash income according to the tax laws operating within your country. However, there is no problem in educating yourself about tax to legally benefit your business and to obtain the maximum tax refunds at the end of each financial year.

One of the most important people in your business is your accountant. Be sure to research your accountant and if you already have one, review their performance to ensure they are working for your business's best interest. A good accountant will save you far more in tax than an average accountant could, therefore shop around and find an accountant who you have confidence in and who is willing to know your business almost as good as you do.

Chapter 3

Handling Enquiries

Handling your customer enquiries in the right way is essential to securing bookings for your business. This chapter explores how you can make the most out of your telephone as well as a variety of client contact options including your answering machine message and email.

Making the most of the telephone

Although email is fast becoming a leading means of communication, many people still prefer the personal touch that comes from speaking over the telephone. The humble telephone is one of your most important pieces of communication equipment so it is wise to make the most of it by using the following suggestions.

Obtain a memorable number

Obtaining a phone number with similar or repeat digits is far more memorable for your clients. If you are looking at upgrading to a new number or if you require a new number for your practice, be sure to contact your phone exchange to see what is possible. In many cases a special request for repeat numbers will incur a higher fee, but in some cases you may be able to obtain a number with repeat digits which an old business has dropped without incurring a special number fee. Phone numbers with repeat numbers or with a rhythm when spoken will be more frequently recalled by your current and future clients.

For example, the number (08) 8855 8855 is far easier to recall than (08) 8435 2956. If you have the option of purchasing an existing number, consider the previous business who owned it. It can be a major problem to receive calls for something other than your business day in and day out.

When I established my practice I called the telephone exchange and requested a search for repeat digits. To my surprise the number (08) 9335 1111 was available. I said I'd take it straight away and have kept it ever since. These days I have it as a back up to my toll free number. I often receive positive comments about the number when dealing with clients and businesses alike.

There are of course some numbers you should not choose. I would advise any natural therapist to avoid phone numbers that have other connotations associated with them. There may be a few reasons why the phone number ending with 666 is readily available.

1800 and 1300 numbers

Toll-free numbers are another option which you may wish to consider. With a toll free number, your clients bear no expense when calling you, which can be an added incentive to do business with you. However, unless you have a large turnover in clients and wish to support this constant flow, then you may not be able to justify the monthly fees as well as paying for all of your clients' calls. Other problems associated with toll free numbers can be when your friends and family hear of the fact that you have a free call number, they might start using your friendly service at your expense. With local rate numbers, the caller only pays for a local call so they suit interstate callers. If you operate a business locally then this option may not suit your business.

How to handle all the calls

Most telephone landlines and mobile networks can offer a voicemail service for callers to leave a message if your phone is engaged or if it is switched off, so that you pick up the message at your convenience. When your phone is really running hot (perhaps from implementing some of the suggestions in this book) you might consider a messaging service so that missed calls can be taken by a person at a telephone bureau. This way your prospective clients can speak to someone who will take their message. Nothing beats the human touch that comes from speaking to a person rather than a recorded message or answering machine.

I'll get back to you!

Let's face it, we all prefer to talk to the person we are calling and when we hear the words on an answering machine, "Your call is important to us", we can't help but think that if it really was that important, they might be there to answer the phone. Unless you have the option of a receptionist or secretary for those working from an established premises, there are a few options for your clients to leave a message.

These include the following:

Answering machines

If you are in business and do not have a way for your clients to leave a message, then it is likely that you will not be in business for very long. Nothing is as frustrating as having no option to leave a message when you call a business.

In the case where you have an answering machine, then careful consideration should be made to your message. If you are not available to be there to answer the phone, then your answering machine message will be your new clients' first impression.

Therefore your message should sound positive, lively and friendly.

Here is an example which you might find useful:

"Hello, you've reached (XXX your name) from (XXX state your business name). I am taking another call right now or giving someone a treatment. However I'm not far away and will get back

to you. Please leave your name and phone number, slowly and clearly, after the tone and I will be happy to return your call just as soon as I can. Thanks for your call and have a great day! BEEP!

Once you have recorded your message, call yourself from another phone and listen to yourself. Do you sound like someone you would like to receive a treatment from?

You can also ask some friends to call your number and listen to your message. Ask for constructive feedback then fine tune your message until it feels and sounds right. If they are real friends, they will be able to tell you honestly what they think of your message.

Getting your message to sound right with variation in your voice is also important. You don't want to sound like you are reading a shopping list when you record your message so remember to make it lively and interesting. You might even wish to write your message greeting down and record it several times until it sounds just right.

One thing I would avoid is pre-recorded or amusing messages which many mobile phone companies now use. This conveys the wrong image of you and your business. Although your clients may think you have a sense of humour, they simply won't take you seriously.

Message bank

Another option is to obtain a message bank service from your telephone service provider. This means that when you are talking to someone else, the person calling can leave a message on your message bank. This way you will not miss any calls. Again, make your message positive, lively and friendly. If your client encounters an engaged signal, they will more likely not bother to call you again or will seek out another therapist, so a message bank is a must for your business.

Call waiting

Call waiting is another less attractive option which you may consider, although some people find the interruption annoying. This is when you are talking to a client and if someone else is trying to get through, *BEEP, BEEP!* can be heard interrupting your conversation.

The downside of this service is that when you hear the *BEEP, BEEP*, you might be tempted to put your client on hold while you tend to something "more important" by saying: *"Can I just put you on hold whilst I see who that is?"* Meanwhile, your client, whose time is precious to them and whose business is precious to you, has been put on hold, having to listen to elevator music.

Please do not do this to your clients. When you say: *"Can I just put you on hold whilst I see who that is?"*, it says to your client that this other person who is interrupting your call is far more important than they are. Nothing devalues your client like taking someone else's call. If they wanted to be put on hold they could call their telephone, mobile, power, gas companies, internet service provider, or any big business to receive bad service. Don't join the same ranks. Keep it personal and friendly and you will earn your clients' respect and patronage.

If you use call waiting, then take the *BEEP* as an advisory to wrap up your call neatly and dial back the number that just tried to get through.

Internet and email

Making bookings via email is becoming more and more common these days. If you advertise your email address you should be sure to create an email which reflects your business's positive message. Every time a client emails you, they are getting a positive re-enforcement that you can benefit them. So choose an email address which reflects your service.

Some examples of email addresses that communicate the benefits of a service might be:

betterback@serviceprovider.com
feelbetternow@serviceprovider.com
healingforyou@serviceprovider.com

If you advertise email as a point of contact be sure to check your email regularly – and by this I mean morning and evening, or at the very least once a day. If someone emails you they want to hear from you as soon as possible. Email is not that different from a phone call. So if you can respond to your emails with speed and efficiency, your clients will feel they are important and respected.

When you send a reply, then your future email correspondence should include an email signature. An email signature means at the end of each email you send, an automatic signature of your contact details, as well as listing benefits of your service or client testimonials. You can even add your company logo to each email by following email program software.

Alternatively you may wish to include a compelling call to action headline or special offer. Remember to make it relevant, memorable and engaging.

Lastly always include your clinic's address, your clinic's phone or your practitioner mobile number, your email and your website information and ensure these are active embedded links in the signature of every email you send – not just sent as one-off information that can be lost in an inbox. This way anyone reading the email can access your information at a glance from your most recent email without having to look for it elsewhere. Your clients need to be able to find your vital booking information easily so this needs to be present on every email signature. Business cards can be lost, but most people keep email in their inbox for years.

For those practitioners reading this who do not have an email account or who are not internet savvy, or who have a fear of technology, then my advice is to get informed. In the last five years we have seen an enormous increase in the use of email. If you are not keen on computers take a short course on basic internet skills. In a matter of one hour, you'll be surfing the net and sending emails. If you're not online, you're not in business so make this a priority if you have not taken this important step already.

If you do not have an email account, you can get email accounts online for free. This means you can also access your email anywhere in the world (provided you can get internet access). So when you are holidaying you can drop into any internet café, sip a latte and check your bookings.

Just visit one of the following free email services to get started:

www.gmail.com
www.hotmail.com
www.yahoo.com

Once you have decided on your free email provider simply click on the sign up email account button, follow the prompts and you'll be on your way. It usually takes about two minutes of your time and if you're not internet savvy, don't worry, setting up these accounts are idiot proof.

Turning an enquiry into a booking

Once you are over the hurdle of having clients call you, the next thing is to turn those enquiries into bookings. Just because someone calls to make an enquiry does not necessarily guarantee a sale. In fact the conversion rate from enquiry to booking is estimated to be less than 10%. Make sure the way you answer their enquiry puts them at ease and brings them in.

Think of it like a person walking into a clothing store and they are looking around. Does this mean that they will make a purchase? It is largely what you have to offer that will determine whether they walk out with nothing or a suit, shoes and three ties.

If you are lucky, some people will already be convinced they wish to use your service and will want to book a time with you when they call. Others will want to know several things and will ask many questions before making a commitment. The thing to remember is that if they are still asking questions, they are still interested.

These are some of the more frequently asked questions made by people making enquiries.

How much?

This is without a doubt the first question on most peoples' minds and is one of the most motivating reasons for anyone taking the step to booking a treatment.

When your future client asks you how much, don't just blurt the price straight away. Instead tell them what they will get for their money first. You might say, *"Can I explain to you what is involved with the treatment so you know what you are paying for?"* Then tell them the fee and add value to what you are offering by telling them about your special offer. For example: *"We also have a special offer, where if you pay in advance for three treatments, your third one is free, so you actually save $50.00".*

In this example your future client will probably now be thinking more about saving $50 over the actual per treatment price.

Will it work?

We all want to make sure that if we are parting with money that it will be worth it. We usually seek recommendations from others who have benefited. This is a real opportunity to tell this person how your therapy can benefit them. Use real life examples and explain how your therapy can benefit them. When we use personal examples it adds credibility, this is why customer testimonials have such power because they help to dissolve any risk for the buyer.

What are your qualifications?

This is another common question which addresses your credibility. This is your opportunity to share with the person your experience and to instill confidence in them that what you are offering can really benefit them. Do your best to re-direct the conversation back to them and what you can do for them. Of course, you should always answer all questions truthfully and never lie about your qualifications in order to impress them. For example, you might say that you have been doing your therapy for x number of years and have successfully treated dozens of people with the same complaint.

When can I receive a treatment?

When someone makes a booking they will want it when it suits them or as close to their chosen time as is humanly possible. If you are busy you can focus on the popularity of your treatments so that they are left with the impression that you are very sought after and must be very good. When someone suggests a time, don't give them a 'no' if this time is not available, but offer an opening. For example, you might say: *"We are already booked at that time but I do have an opening on Friday at 4pm for 2 hours. We could fit you in for a treatment at this time and if you wish we could throw in a complimentary 30 minute pamper bonus"*.

Where are you located?

One of the common questions when someone is considering a booking is the location and whether parking will be an issue. If you happen to be in a location which has easy parking options you should feature this in your telephone conversations and on all your advertising materials. People look for convenience and getting to and from your place of practice can mean the difference in whether someone makes a booking. It can be a deal breaker. Featuring the ease of parking or that there is free customer parking can be used to your advantage. Making the whole experience as hassle free as possible removes risk for the customer.

If you have a venue which is difficult when it comes to parking, but offers a good public transport system, rather than bringing attention to the parking problems, feature the excellent and easy public transport system. For example tell them it is convenient for commuters, *'Just two minutes stroll from Kings Street station'*. Notice how I used the word 'stroll' rather than 'walk'. It implies a relaxing journey. I'd rather stroll than walk any day.

In short, feature the ease of parking or public transport and try not to bring attention to negatives with relation to your business, unless you can use this to your advantage.

On the other hand, if they mention they will be coming by car, and you know the parking is awkward outside the clinic, it could save a lot of stress on the day if you give them a good tip for on-street parking – even if it is 10 minutes stroll away, so that they can arrive for the appointment on time and not too fraught.

Answering questions with confidence

When your prospective clients ask you questions (and they will), you should welcome their interest and answer their questions directly and with confidence. Coming across uncertain or avoiding a question will immediately make your prospective client feel suspicious. Most people make decisions based on their emotions, so it is best to be genuinely friendly and honest in all your communications. The more natural we can be when answering questions the more likely we will be to secure business.

If this is not your natural forte then it is a great idea to write a list of questions that you think your clients may ask, such as the ones listed in the previous section and then write out the answers and highlighting the key benefits distinctly. You might even wish to highlight the key benefits with bullets. This way you can quickly identify the key benefits at a glance.

A great way to practise answering questions with confidence is to role-play with a friend. You could even pretend to have a telephone conversation. Here you present your friend with a list of questions which they ask you at random and you do your best to answer these in a clear and friendly manner. Allow your answers to be spontaneous and for new questions to arise out of the conversation.

Another way to practice is to rehearse questions and answers to your self in the mirror. This might feel a little strange at first but it is a great way to practice; plus the only audience you need to please is yourself. You can also repeat this process and record your self then play back the recording to hear how you sound. This is a great way to hear how you sound as well as take note of adjustments where necessary.

When customers phone you to make enquiries, they very often call for the basic facts. New customers make 'scan' calls in just the same way they scan a magazine or the internet. In reality you have about 30 seconds to retain and keep a prospective client's interest. Do your best to answer their questions quickly and in such a way that you not only answer their questions but offer solutions to their problems as efficiently as possible.

Talking with clients and rebooking

What do you do when it is time for your client to leave? Here you have the opportunity for repeat business and most customers will welcome suggestions (if they were happy with your service) and generally expect some follow up. If your client could benefit from further treatments then to encourage a rebooking is certainly a benefit to both yourself as well as to the client.

If, for example, you are a massage therapist, then discuss with your client what benefits were derived after your treatment and welcome any feedback. Before they leave suggest what areas could benefit from further work and suggest a treatment plan.

Now at this point your client has a choice to say yes or no. However, by simply changing the way you ask the question can give your client every opportunity to say yes to another session. Of course your client has free will and can still say no, all you are doing is providing them with every reason to say yes.

To ensure your client has every opportunity to rebook there are three things which are helpful. The first is to recap once again the benefits of your therapy and what has been achieved as a result of your treatment. The second is to describe what future benefits can be achieved. The third is to offer them the opportunity to book a treatment series where they will receive a discount or a bonus gift.

Three cards are better than one

At the end of your session whether your client wishes to rebook or not, offer them three of your business cards when leaving. Let them know that most of your bookings come from word of mouth advertising and that you'd really appreciate it if they passed your cards onto family and friends. You may be surprised that most people will happily do this. You can mention that if they enjoyed the treatment that it would really help to let others know. Three business cards (instead of one) will usually end up in their pocket or hand bag which is the perfect place when they go out next time with friends.

One sentence has tremendous referral business that keeps on working. Just ask.

Chapter 4

Establishing your Unique Selling Proposition (USP)

In this chapter, I will share with you the benefits of establishing your unique selling proposition or 'USP'. Let's face it you are probably not the only natural therapist in your town. There is always competition and people have lots of choices. How will you make yourself stand out from the crowded natural therapist marketplace? You need to find an edge, something that makes you and your business unique. What makes what you do enticing, different? How will you flag down your prospects over your competitors?

The answer lies in establishing your USP.

Now you may be thinking that what you offer is basically the same service as any other practitioner in your field, and this may even be the case. You may even have had the same training and came out of the same natural therapy college. How will you make yourself stand out as offering something truly unique?

You do this by creating your Unique Selling Proposition or U.S.P. The first thing you need to recognise is what you do is unique and unlike anyone else. Nobody is a carbon copy of another, aside from the outer methods you may use in your consultations, what is unique, is you. By this I am not suggesting that you become your USP. What I do want you to acknowledge is that you are the one who is responsible for creating something unique about what you do.

Once you have established your USP, you need to make this message clear and concise and deliver this message across all your promotional materials. Whether you base your USP on your name or business name, in effect you are establishing a new brand in the market place. Think about how other businesses have used their USP's to make themselves stand out from their competitors.

Creating your USP is the very thing which illustrates the key benefits you offer over your competition. Your USP is designed to immediately communicate. For the most part, many natural therapists neglect to create a USP and instead they simply follow the advertising that others have already done. You need only flick through a new age magazine and you'll see the same kind of ads, saying basically the same thing as well as looking the same.

I call these *'name, rank and serial number'* ads. The ad is usually the same with the name of the therapy or therapist (name), their qualifications or modalities offered (rank), and a contact number (serial number). Some ads will also feature a photo of the practitioner or their logo. Rarely is there a reason or set of reasons why they can solve your problems. Avoid becoming yet another formula advertiser. Make yourself stand out from the rest.

For example, you might be a Naturopath. You could advertise that you offer Naturopathy consultations but so do all the other Naturopaths. An example of a USP could be a Naturopath who specialises in weight control and offers weight loss solutions. The USP in this case might be: *ABC Naturopathy – the natural weight loss solution.*

Perhaps you are a Hypnotherapist. Instead of advertising Hypnotherapy in a general manner, you could focus on a specific target market. For example, you may specialise in treating people who want to quit smoking. Your USP might read: *Quit Smoking for Life! - Hypnotherapy Specialist.*

Whatever it is that you do, if you specialise your therapy to a specific target market and advertise in this way you will no longer be: Bob Smith, Hypnotherapist. You will be *Bob Smith – 'Quit Smoking for Life Specialist'– guaranteed to help you quit for life or your first consultation is free.* In this example, you move from being just a Hypnotherapist who does all kinds of treatments to someone who is now a specialist in assisting people quit smoking, plus you offer a solid risk-free guarantee.

It is also important to recognise that some natural therapies are very similar in nature so your USP may come down to finding an edge with unique service or your unique personality. With any of your advertising or marketing you need to communicate to your potential customers that you and/or your service are the best and the only choice they should consider.

What is your USP? If you don't have one, you need to create one, for it enables you to position yourself in the marketplace and celebrates what makes you and your services unique and appealing. Without one you remain just another therapist who remains largely unsuccessful, another name, rank and serial number advertisement in the local paper.

How to create your USP

Your USP should avoid the three following mistakes:

1. It should not contain vague terminology or language which could apply to almost all therapies and which the average person will not understand anyway.
2. It should not be based on features such as the latest equipment or that you have qualifications in such and such or that you have recently renovated your clinic.
3. It should not take longer than 5 seconds to communicate your message.

Your USP should be based on the three following golden rules:

1. It should communicate clearly to your target specific audience.
2. It should concisely identify the customer's problem and offer the solution.
3. It should be make you or your business unique and clearly set

you apart from your competitors.

When selecting a USP for your business, identify your key benefits and what makes your practice unique. It should cater for your target audience, solve a general problem and make you stand out.

Let's look at each point in more detail:

The target audience

In identifying your target audience you may well think that this applies to just about everyone. For example, if you are a massage therapist you might well assume that just about anyone would appreciate and indeed be in need of a massage. However, the whole point in identifying your target audience is to offer a specialty in order to attract these target clients. Not just massage but specialty massage. For example, you might focus on pregnancy massage so in this case this is your target audience.

Offering a solution

Following on from our example of pregnancy massage the solution we offer is of benefit for both mother and baby. A pregnant mother is having to cope with all of her body's changes; the stress of having to carry the additional load, especially in the third term of pregnancy; as well as all the hopes and fears that accompany a huge life transition.

So what is the solution? Is it making the mother more comfortable and relaxed, or is it more than this? You need to get inside your client's head and think what it is that they really want from your service.

Your unique angle

Finding your unique angle that will enable you to stand out from your fellow practitioners is essential for business success. For our pregnancy massage therapist, this may extend to a relaxation massage treatment tailored to the individuals needs creating a relaxing atmosphere for the mother which also means a happy baby.

Your U.S.P. might be:

'Mother to be', Pregnancy Massage Specialists – Gently nurturing you and your baby through pregnancy.

Price based USP's

A word of advice on making your USP price based is that most practitioners who compete by being the cheapest will not stay in business for very long. There will always be someone else who is willing to offer their service that little bit cheaper than you. Fighting the price war makes you and your business look cheap, amateurish and even questionable. When it comes to natural therapies most customers are prepared to pay a fair price, the standard going rate, or even a little extra if they know they will receive a quality treatment.

If you went to a doctor for open heart surgery you probably would not select your physician because they were the cheapest in town. You also wouldn't select a lawyer because they were the cheapest if you had a great deal to lose. There is some perceived truth to the saying: *'If you pay peanuts, you get monkeys'.*

The same applies to the complementary health field. It is better to offer a slightly more expensive service and offer something unique. Your customers will be happy to pay more when they know they will be receiving something special.

Discounting can see the end of your business. Instead I suggest you create some great special offers that stand out. Up-selling on the other hand does just the opposite. See: *Up-Selling verses Discounting* in Chapter 7 for more.

Why not have a go at writing your USP now. Take a few moments to fill in your USP.

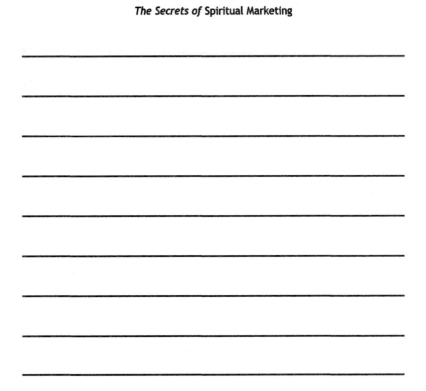

How to sell yourself

Have you noticed that whenever you meet someone new that somewhere along the line the inevitable question will be asked, *'By the way, what do you do for a living?'*. How would you answer this question as a natural therapist?

If you are a massage therapist you'd probably say, *'I'm a massage therapist'*. But how little do you think this communicates to your new acquaintance? As soon as you label a therapy by name you limit the therapy to the other person's pre-conceived ideas about the therapy. They will have in their mind their own idea of what a massage therapist is and you would have told them nothing about, 'what you do and how you can benefit them'. All you would have told them is the name of the modality you practice.

By taking the same question from a *Spiritual Marketing* perspective, the answer is completely different. When asked the same question, someone who utilises the opportunity to sell themselves and what they do for a living might respond by saying:

"You know how you can get stressed out from time to time and get tense muscles? Well, what I do is help people to facilitate a natural unwinding process which leaves them feeling re-energized and self-empowered. I utilise a numbers of techniques to release the body's tension in a gentle and pain free way."

How do you think the person would respond to your answer? The person would probably be very interested to find out more about this amazing treatment, wouldn't you?

When you describe the benefits of your service, rather than just giving it to them straight out, you develop interest. This approach immediately captivates your audience and they can't help but ask for more information.

The idea with selling yourself is to paint a picture of what you do which illustrates the benefits of your modality and communicates these directly to your client. You effectively identity a common problem and offer a solution to their problem through your conversation.

You may want to pause a moment from reading and imagine being asked the question, *'What do you do for a living?'* How would you respond using this method?

Would you simply tell them your qualifications or titles? The answer of course is no as this would only offer your interested enquirer information about your credentials and give them no further clue as to what you do and how you can help them.

They want to know whether what you do can benefit them in any way. This comes under the WIIFM principle, which stands for What's In It For Me. If you're not describing to the person 'what is in it for me', you will lose their interest straight away.

Take a few moments to list as many benefits you can think of when your clients receives a treatment. Include how these benefits eliminate stress or pain. Also list all of the beneficial outcomes from your treatment, such as more relaxed, sleeping better and the like.

Stop reading now and fill in the benefits below.

Key benefits from my treatments/therapy:

1. _____

2. _____

3. _____

4. _____

5. _____

6. _____

7. _____

8. _____

9. _____

10. _____

Once you have determined all of the benefits of what you do, narrow these down to the top three benefits. Identify the top three benefits now.

1. _____

2. _____

3. _____

These are your 'Gold benefits' and you can tie these into your response when answering the question: 'what do you do for a living?'.

Some helpful hints when composing your response is to have these presented in two parts. The first identities the person's problem and the second, offers the solution to the problem.

For example, you might say in reply: *"You know how you can get stressed out from time to time and get tense muscles?"* and then list the problem or problems that you feel the person will relate to. This paints a picture in their mind and they will already be thinking: *"Yeah, I can sure relate to that"*. In this way you captivate their interest.

Then you offer a solution. Here you say: *"What I do is..."* and then offer the solution to their problem. Suddenly you move on from being a massage therapist, healer or naturopath to someone who *is* the answer to their problems.

Do you think they will want to know more? You bet they will! The reason is that you have identified their problems and offered solutions to their problems.

Seven reasons

Now that we have identified your USP and the key benefits of your practice in relation to the customer's question: 'WIIFM', we will now explore seven key reasons to make a purchase with you.

It is said that if you can present seven good reasons why someone should part with their hard-earned money, you will be more likely to secure their business.

In the following table you can list seven benefits of your treatments.

You might include:

- Some of the health and relaxation benefits.
- How relaxing the treatment is.
- Your sound experience and anything else which makes your service of benefit to your client.

Remember your client is asking in their mind, *'What's in it for me?'*

Listing these seven good reasons can become part of all your promotional materials by including this list at the end of your emails; on letterheads; business cards; client invoices; and, press advertising to name a few. People want results and they want to know it is safe and that it can improve their health and well-being.

Stop reading now and get to work on creating your seven good reasons.

1. _____

2. _____

3. _____

4. _____

5. _____

6. _____

7. _____

Chapter 5

Establishing your Website

In this chapter, we will map out all the necessary information you need to know about creating a website that is both a functional resource and powerful marketing tool. In addition to this we will explore how to register a domain name; create your online content; explore what you should add; and, what you should avoid on your website.

We will also explore establishing an online shop; various payment options; registering with search engines; reciprocal links; advertising banners; email databases; online consultations; and web seminars.

To begin we need to consider the benefits of having a website and the reasons are many. Having a professionally designed and well oiled website provides a valuable resource for your clients and presents a professional edge to your practice.

First and foremost it is important to know that it is not necessary to spend thousands to establish a professional looking website. Nor is it necessary to feature dozens of pages or have fancy flash graphics on your site to be effective. On the other hand it is not recommended that you build your own website unless of course you have professional training in website production and graphic design. If you opt for a very basic site with little attention to the design and functionality you will present an unprofessional image to your clients. It will simply look home made which is fine if you are making jam for charity but when it comes to websites a professional look is very important.

Having a website provides a practical way for your clients to research you and your services before they call or email you. You may be surprised just how many people make buying decisions via the internet over conventional methods such as press advertising or other non-electronic media. In many cases, your clients will come across your website via email advertising, your business card, or a classified or press advertisement. Your website is perhaps even more important than your phone number.

Before we look into the design and content of your website you first need a name. Just in the same way you may have registered a business or company name to trade under so it is that you need to have a website domain so that your clients can search your site on the internet and locate your website.

Registering a domain name

Securing a domain name is a relatively simple task and there are many options. My suggestion is that you go with a domain registration company that is in your own country and check to see that you can actually call them if required.

When selecting a name for your website you will probably need to have a few options up your sleeve as your desired name may or may not already have been taken by someone else. This is particularly the case when you are choosing a '*.com*' domain which denotes a website with an international flavour.

If, for example, if you are living in the United Kingdom then your website will end in '*.co.uk*' or if you are living in Australia it will end with '*.com.au*'. There are other options to these as you will discover when registering your domain name online. Further alternatives include: *.tv .us .info .net .org .biz .mobi .ws .name .ag .am .at.*

The list goes on and on.

When registering your domain you may find it easier to find your name if you choose to have the name ending with the country web code.

Although '*.com*' and '*.net*' are the most widely preferred options perhaps the most important is the name you select. What comes after '*www.*' is the name which best represents your business. For example, if you are a Reflexology practitioner, a memorable domain name might be one of the following domain names:

www.treatyourfeet.com
www.healingyoursoles.com
www.solefeeling.com

Alternatively if you are a massage therapist, then you might choose a domain name which represents the benefits of your therapy. For example:

www.backtobalance.com
www.mostlymassage.com
www.massageworks.com

Another recommendation is not to make your domain name too long.

An example of a domain that is too long would be: www.southsydneyholistichealingmassageforthebodyandsoul.com.au.

Every time someone wants to visit your site they will have to type in this long name, which in web terms is a few too many seconds too long. Plus there will be many more chances for the customer to make typing errors.

If you have not already secured your domain name some recommended websites for domain registration include:

www.godaddy.com
www.planetdomain.com

www.australianwebsites.com.au
www.australiacheapdomains.com.au
www.net2.co.uk
www.ukreg.com
www.MyDomain.com

Happy domain hunting!

Creating your website

Once you have secured your domain name you will need to be clear on your website production budget as well as the content for your website.

The best way to get started is to search the internet through a search engine such as www.google.com and type into the search bar the names of your modalities to get an idea of what is currently out there.

Once you have found a variety of websites that you like (and I suggest you take your time to research this) you can start to make notes and draw simple maps of how you think the layout of your website could be. Take note of the features that you would like added and remember the more animation and dynamic drop down menus you desire as apposed to a more static looking website, the higher the price will be.

It is important to take your time to plan your website as the more of an idea you can have as to the content, look and feel of your website, the better prepared you will be when selecting a website designer to construct the website.

As for the content, (in other words the information for your website) it is ideal to have this in an electronic format so that it can be easily cut and pasted into the website as per your directions when working with a web designer.

You will also need to consider how many pages you will need. More simple websites feature: *About Us*; *Contact Us*; *Bookings* or a *Registration* Page; *Frequently Asked Questions*; and, an *About Us* page.

A more complex site may also include such headings as: *Online Shop; Links; Forum; Newsletter Registration; Search this Site* facility; *Add to Favourites* page; *Blog; Media Room; Send to a Friend* page; *Client Testimonials; Guest Book; Special Offers; Privacy Policy; Site Map; Resources; Downloads; Articles* and *Press Releases.*

It is not necessary to have all of these options as some websites are hundreds of pages long. If you can convey clearly what you offer and persuade customers to book with you, you have succeeded.

Generally, the higher the price for the service or product, the more you need to tell to sell. If you are offering a workshop that costs thousands of dollars then a few sentences will probably not convince your audience. On the other hand if you are simply selling a treatment then a few paragraphs may be enough. Generally, depending upon the topic and the level of interest your customers may be happy to read through all the pages listed on your website. For those who just want the basic information they will also be able to get this if you make your content easy to read.

When it comes to images, your web designer may have access to stock photography or you may have your own collection of images (which is preferable as most stock photography looks like stock photography). Whatever the case may be, be sure to have copyright on the images you use and not simply borrow these from other websites you like. Fines can be hefty for copyright infringement.

Once you have your plans, you can use the internet to locate a web designer in your area. It is best to choose a web designer you can visit in person as you will probably need to visit them on a number of occasions in the construction phase.

Most website designers will be happy to meet you for a no obligation introductory session from which a basic template can be generated to give you an indication of where they are headed with the project. It is also ideal to set a quote for the website upfront to avoid an ever escalating fee for the website's construction. You can easily spend thousands of dollars with no set quote.

When selecting a web designer, ask them to send you *links* to examples of the websites they have produced and ask them to give you an indication on how much these websites cost so you have a comparison that aligns to your website.

I recommend obtaining three separate quotes initially from three different web designers. You may be surprised just how vastly different quotes can be. This is not to say that you should opt for the cheapest quote as there may be a reason for the low price. Do your due diligence and be happy with your web designer, it will be the grounds for a long term business relationship.

Website content and things to consider

Once you have found a web designer you have confidence in, there are a number things that you should add to your site to maximise your marketing efforts.

Likewise, there are a number of things you should avoid. In Seth Godin's book *The Big Red Fez – how to make any web site better*, he gives several helpful insights of what works and what fails to hit the mark with website design, content and functionality.

Here is a brief summary of some of the ideas presented in *The Big Red Fez*. These include:

- Show me the money.
- Keep it simple.
- Page loading…
- Make it easy for me.
- Remember me.
- Make it legible.

- Test, Test, Test.
- Say thank you.
- Make it easy to share.
- Offer me something special.
- Offer me [more].
- Say sorry.
- Check for typos and grammar.

Show me the money

Show me the money is the principle that when a person lands on your home page their attention is immediately drawn to one place in particular. What that place is depends on what you wish to stand out the most on your home page. Perhaps it is a special offer, a free e-newsletter or free information report to tell your customers about your products or services. When you and your designer create your website you should determine what the most important items are for you. Illustrate this with good design and navigation and you will be able to influence how someone moves around your website.

You can do much to assist your net surfer to catch the right wave simply with the use of clever design or an attention-grabbing headline which compels the reader to click wherever it is that you want them to go. You need to remember that everyone who visits your website is just one click away from leaving so make your content fresh and engaging and give the customer the information they are looking for with sound navigation and innovative design. Your web designer will be able to assist you in creating a logical layout to drive the net surfer around your website to the pages which ultimately translate (if done well) into a purchase.

Keep it simple

Have you ever been online filling out a web form which ends up taking forever? If you keep your web forms simple and avoid endless drop down menus to select a country for example, you will do your customers a favour. The trick to a great website is to make it seamlessly smooth for the person buying, whether it is booking a massage treatment or buying a product, the bare minimum of personal information the better. The last thing you want to do is waste your customer's time with unnecessary information and endless typing.

Page loading...

A website should load fast and this includes your introduction. A great deal of money is spent on websites that are trying too hard to look like television. Have you ever come across a website that requires you to download a program just to open it? Other sites take up to a minute to load or more, and feature a page loading sign that counts up from 0% to 100%. In the time it takes to load the page the customer has already made the one click back taking their business elsewhere. Flash graphics and start pages waste time for your customers and cost the earth to produce. The less clicks to get to the information required, the better off you'll be plus more customers will stay on your website for longer. I recommend you save your money for the website's content and not on unnecessary flash content which takes ages to load.

Make it easy for me

Making it easy for me means, being able to easily navigate through the website. You can do this by utilising a logical search facility as well as offering clear navigation menus. These should preferably be at the top or left hand side of your website as well as offering hot links at the bottom of each page. Include a back to top on each page which links to the top of the page plus back and next buttons for easy navigation throughout the website.

Remember me

Whenever you sign into a website for a free newsletter or to establish an account you will need to give your name and email address to register. When you do this make sure your web designer can record this information so that each time you go back to the website the site remembers who you are.

I love www.amazon.com for this very reason. Each time I visit the site it says: *"Hello, Lawrence Ellyard. We have recommendations for you"*. Don't you feel so much more appreciated when people remember your name? Why should it be any different when surfing on your website?

Make it legible

Whatever you do, ensure you use type which is both legible and large enough so that people with smaller computer monitors or bad eyesight can actually read your webpage. Avoid background colours or coloured type which clash or are hard to read. The idea is that you want to make reading your website a pleasure for the person reading it, not a chore. Remember if it is too small, too hard to read or just plain ugly, your possible customer is one click away from your competitors.

Test, Test, Test

Test your website to ensure that your web designer has not made fatal errors. There is nothing as off putting as clicking to visit a particular page only to encounter an error page or worse the wrong page. It reflects poorly on you and your practice. Nobody knows your website as well as you do, so be sure to check your website on a monthly basis that all links are working and go where they are required to go. Also, make it your business to check the work of your web designer to ensure they have understood and executed your requests. Do not assume that your web designer does not make errors with links. Test your site before it goes live and get others to check it to see if errors have been made.

Say thank you

Whatever happened to manners? If you went to a shop and made a purchase, do you think you would feel warm and fuzzy if the shop assistant said nothing to you once you'd paid? A simple *'thank you for your booking'* or *'your purchase is greatly appreciated'* is not a lot to ask but so many websites neglect to add this common courtesy.

After you click 'submit', you should be directed to a thank you page where you are thanked for your business as well as being given any important *'what happens next'* information. This may include the terms of being contacted, delivery times or at least the opportunity to continue browsing the website with the click of a button such as *'continue shopping'* or *'click here to go back to home page'*.

Word of mouse

One of the most important buttons on your website is the option to *'send to a friend'*. Here your customers can actively refer you and better still be rewarded for sharing your website with others.

This is what is called: *'Word of Mouse'*. With the click of the mouse, your customers can actively share the benefits of your treatments. Offer incentives to share your website include 'a points system' or a 'referral rewards program'. This feature alone can offer you some of the best *word of mouse* and the added benefit is that it costs you nothing.

If you are utilising a points system you can give your existing customer 100 points every time they actively refer a new customer to you. Once they reach 1000 points they may qualify for a free treatment for example. A referral rewards program works in a similar fashion, here you might give your existing customer a free gift for a certain number of referrals.

Offer me something special

Have you noticed that most retail outlets seem to always have some kind of special or sale? What are you going to offer your customers when they walk through your virtual door? Be sure to offer a discount on making a treatment series or a free gift when making a purchase over a designated amount. Make that offer stand out and give them a reason to buy.

Offer me [more]

On your home page instead of creating so much content that the person will get sore fingers from scrolling down the page endlessly, offer an overview with useful links such as [more] or [read on] so that those who want more information can be linked to a new page with greater detail and those who just want the bare minimum can get the information they need within a few sentences. You'll keep everyone happy this way.

Say sorry

If you make an error such as missing an order or being overly late to reply to an enquiry, say sorry. If it was a huge oversight on your behalf be accountable and offer the customer a small gift as an apology. This is part of offering exceptional customer service. Your goal is to exceed your customers' expectations. When you don't, you are like almost every other business. Stand out and offer exceptional customer service and when you make a mistake, exceed their expectations once more.

For example, I sent out one of my meditation CDs in the post and due to poor handling the case was cracked upon arrival. I had packed it well enough but the postman may have had a bad day. The customer emailed to advise that the case was damaged and requested a replacement case. What I did was to send a new case express post plus a second copy of the CD for free along with an apology note personally signed. It only cost me a few dollars and a small amount of time but in the end I turned a not so happy customer into a customer for life.

Check for typos and grammar

Before you submit your content to your designer to be uploaded to your website, be sure to check your content for typos and grammar. The information presented on your website represents you and should be correct down to the little details. When I am reading a website that is professionally designed and I encounter a spelling mistake or an incorrectly constructed sentence it is a disappointing experience which does not instill a great deal of confidence.

The same goes for website alterations or changes made by your web designer. If you try and do changes and amendments over the telephone your web designer could make some errors in type, so always supply any corrections by email, and ensure the amendments are correctly spelled content via email. Always check and re-check your content. Share your website around to your friends for feedback. A fresh pair of eyes can spot an error faster than someone who has read and re-read the same materials many times.

Now that you are armed with the necessary dos and don'ts, you may also wish to consider the following items to expand your spiritual marketing repertoire.

Establishing an online shop

An additional income source to your natural therapy practice is having your very own online shop. Your consultations or workshops can also be shop items.

In my experience having a designated shopping cart as part of your website provides a great way to up-sell additional products in line with your natural therapy practice. Talk to your web designer about which options may suit your needs and what is possible within your budget. You may wish to keep it simple and only stock a few products or you may wish to open a fully fledged online super-store. Be sure to test your market before you invest a lot of money and time into an online store. Offering a great many products means you will need to have the stock for orders as well as needing space to store the products.

If you do wish to offer an online shop, check for wholesalers who can provide you with a suitable discount for products which you can sell to your clients.

Establish an account where you can pay for your orders on a 30 day account or longer if possible (the longer the better). This will keep your start up costs down and you won't have to pay for the stock advertised on your online shop up front.

Alternatively, you may wish to order from your wholesaler as orders some in. You may encounter, however, that most whole-salers have minimum orders or cannot deliver in an expedient manner. You want to ensure that your customers can get their products fast, so make sure you either advise delivery times in length of days or state the maximum time a customer will have to wait before delivery.

In addition to this you will need to consider freight and packaging for your products. Be sure to cover these costs with orders.

Most online shops charge postage after the purchase of products. For orders over a specific amount you may wish to cover the postage, thus ensuring your customers spend more in order to get the free freight. For example, you may offer a monthly special such as: *"Spend over $100 and we'll freight your order for free"*.

Look into postage / courier delivery costs and consider also if you are prepared to offer international freight or delivery only within your country.

Palpal versus merchant credit card facilities

If you are going to establish an online store you will need to make a decision as to what kind of shopping cart system you wish to obtain. If you do not have merchant facilities where you can process all the major credit cards such as *Mastercard* and *Visa* you may wish to bypass this cost by designating your shopping cart through an outside merchant provider such as *Paypal*. See: www.paypal.com for details.

Having *Paypal* as your payment gateway is considerably cheaper over establishing a private merchant facility. However, *Paypal* does take a percentage of your transactions but even so it can be a more cost effective alternative to having your own fully fledged online merchant facility. One problem I see with *Paypal* is that it communicates that you are not a big enough player and so you require a third party to process your credit card payments. In the end it is a question of turnover. Check with your web designer and discuss which options suit both your needs and your hip pocket.

When it comes to accepting credit cards it is also important to know that *American Express* and *Diners* attract higher percentages over *Visa* and *Mastercard*. You will also need to apply to be a merchant with these two individually where as *Visa* and *Mastercard* can be established through your bank when registering for your merchant account. Contact your local bank for more information about establishing a merchant account and to see if your business qualifies.

Another alternative is not to accept credit cards and only accept cash, cheque, internet banking or postal money orders. The problem is that we are increasingly becoming a credit society (particularly online). Most people do not necessarily carry cash and writing cheques have the possibility of being dis-honoured. Postal money orders cost more for the customer, plus they have to go to the post office to get one. Probably the better option of these is internet banking but, if you really want to shine, credit cards are the way to go.

Registering with search engines

There are a great many websites available on the internet today who will charge you a great deal of money to have your website listed in the top ten on search engines such as www.*google.com*.

In my experience, one of the best ways to improve your ratings in search engines is to make sure you add key words to your internet page descriptions. Your web designer will also have some good advice for structuring and programming your website to increase your exposure and improving your rating on search engines.

Another great way to improve your ratings is to get as many people to visit your website as possible. The more people who visit your site, the higher your rating becomes.

This can be considerably sped up with a high impact website launch that combines emailing to previous clients and advertising through print media where readers will be compelled to visit your site for one of your fantastic offers. Just in the same way an author may do a book launch, launching your website can be an online launch event.

Once you are happy with your website, send it to all of your contacts and ask for feedback. Email, text message or phone your friends and clients. This will get the ball rolling and provide you with valuable tips of how you might improve your website before the official launch.

Reciprocal links

Working hand-in-hand with other businesses using reciprocal links can do a great deal to enhance your practice, your profile, and enable you to stand out in an otherwise overly competitive online marketplace. Reciprocal links are a great way to exchange your domain with other professionals with websites within your industry. It is also a great way to build online communities and strategic alliances.

The more websites your domain is listed with, the greater

your internet presence will be. Select websites that are of a higher profile than your own. The bigger fish naturally have a bigger internet presence and you can get a free ride by having your website listed with some of these websites. For example, if you are a massage therapist, reciprocal link to a massage therapy company who sells massage products online or one of the major massage colleges. If you think outside the box you will find there are many opportunities to increase your internet presence.

In my experience when being approached by other companies for reciprocal links I personally take into consideration the websites that I am exchanging with. My criteria for reciprocal links are three fold:

1. The website must be related to the wellness industry.
2. The website must look professional and be of a high standard.
3. The website must rate well on search engines.

Although I am often approached by a variety of companies for a reciprocal link, very few meet my criteria to be selected. There is no point in listing a site that is not industry related, it makes you look as if you are 'selling out' and will send out a message that you will invite anyone to link sites. This in turn attracts 'spam' and junk mail to your website.

You should be selective and aim for quality sites which will enhance your online profile and offer a mutually beneficial online relationship, which can be further nurtured through strategic alliances. For more on strategic alliances see chapter 12 on networking your business.

Advertising banners

Advertising banners are another way to promote your website and services on other wellness industry websites. In addition to reciprocal links, an advertising banner which is situated on a high profile and well visited website can really improve your website ratings as well as directing new internet traffic to your website.

In order to achieve this ensure your advertising banner is visually engaging and in much the same way as a small space advertisement in a newspaper, your banner must have an immediate and compelling headline to entice the viewer to click on it.

As you can probably relate, when you are surfing the internet, you are not looking for ads but information. If your banner looks like it leads to important information or contains information about a special offer which is too good to pass up you will have a higher success rate than having a fancy image alone which may look interesting but has no compelling call to action.

It matters that people actually take that step to pointing and clicking. It may seem obvious but featuring a click here or click now or read more link which links to your site is essential.

When creating your advertising banner, make sure it communicates instantly because that is about all the time you have to get your message across online. You may wish to use examples from chapter 9 on how to write a great headline as a starting point for your advertising banner.

When submitting your banner advertisement ensure the recipient has your URL (Uniform Resource Location), which is your website domain address. Be sure to test the banner to ensure it works and links correctly to your website.

Email databases

If another practitioner is willing to share links or advertising banners, you may be able to further the friendly relationship to sharing or at least advertising in their email newsletter. In most cases practitioners will not be overly happy to give you their client list. If they do you may have to check the validity of this list as these recipients may have already been subjected to spam from other unauthorised parties.

I cannot stress the importance of making sure you select the right email lists. You want your product or service to hit the mark. Just as there is no point in advertising in Guns and Ammo Magazine as a Naturopath, the same goes for not advertising online with email newsletters that miss the correct target market.

If you can advertise your services through a reliable e-list (perhaps for a small fee), if the list is extensive and is aimed at your target audience it may be money well spent. A way around paying a small fee is to offer an exchange for a mention on your e-list.

When composing the script for the advertisement, make it clear and easy to follow. If you can arrange for the practitioner who owns the e-list to give you a personal endorsement about your services you will also obtain a better response. This is because it is like a trusted friend making a recommendation about your services.

Online consultations

Have you given any thought as to how you may be able to translate some of your services electronically? In addition to your regular consultations, you may be able to give follow up consultations online in the form of email correspondence or live chat such as MSN (www.msn.com) or Skype (www.skype.com).

You may be able to offer one-on-one scheduled appointments using a mounted pod cast from your monitor or utilise other live portals for your follow-up consultations via the internet. Because the internet is global you may also be able to give consultations in other cities or even other countries. It bears thinking about.

There could be a whole world of untapped business waiting for you. Internet consultations mean you don't have to go to work, you can choose your hours and have the added bonus of working from the privacy of your home.

Webinars (online webcam seminars)

Just in the same way as you may consider offering online consultations, you may choose to offer workshops in your chosen field online. A webinar is an online seminar where you present in real time a seminar linked to webcam with recipients who have already paid online to attend via secure log in. Alternatively, you can present a pre-recorded seminar that customers subscribe to and download for viewing at a time that is more suitable. There is unlimited scope for online classes, consultations and downloadable e materials. If marketed correctly with the right incentives you can open the doors to new business just by working from home.

Chapter 6

Your Promotional Materials

In this chapter we will explore a variety of tools you can utilise to promote your practice, including: business cards; advertising on invoices; email; offering a free report; e newsletters; featuring client testimonials; and, gift vouchers to name a few. We will also explore some general guidelines for graphic design and how to go about printing your promotional materials.

Business cards – your mobile advertisement

Every time you meet someone new, it is an opportunity to network your business. This does not need to be aggressive networking which many people resent, especially if they are being canvassed to join a Network Marketing Company or MLM (Multi-Level Marketing). In all but a few cases when you meet someone new, people will eventually come to the question of what you do for a living. This can be an opportunity to explain what you do which includes the key benefits of your practice. The thing is you never know just how often you will encounter an opportunity to network your business and this is why you should always have at least a few business cards on you at all times.

Most people think of a business card simply as a place to have your contact information but business cards can be so much more than this. Your business card is your mobile advertisement. Your business card, although small, is for many the only item of yours to remember you by, so spare no expense in utilising both the front and back of your business card.

Some people prefer to keep their business cards rather 'Zen' and simply offer their name and phone number. The thing is that the more you tell, the more likely you are to sell. Although you are short on space with the average business cards dimensions being 90mm x 55mm, you can actually fit a considerable amount of information in this small space.

Your business card should feature at least the following items:

- Your name.
- Your company or business name.
- The services or treatments you offer.
- Your qualifications / the letters after your name.
- Your phone or mobile number.
- Your email address.
- Your website address.

You know all this. But did you know it can also feature:

- Your USP (unique selling proposition).
- Your professional affiliations and memberships.
- A client testimonial.
- A compelling headline.

Perhaps the most important feature of your business card is the compelling heading. This features the key benefits or solution to your client's problem. I know what you are thinking, that sounds like a lot of information, but with the right design and use of space you can create a card that really is a mobile advertisement.

Once you have created your business cards along with a talented graphic designer (who by the way may suggest you don't add this much to a card) you can arrange to have these printed. The difference in price between printing 500 and 2500 cards is not as much as you might think.

If you have a great deal of cards you will also be mentally more liberal when handing these around to your clients. Remember to offer your clients or anyone new at least three of your business cards and ask them to share them around.

You can also leave small piles of cards at health centres, cafes and the like. Remember to ask permission from the businesses to leave your cards otherwise they might end up in the bin the same day.

The golden rule is *the more you tell, the more you sell.*

Keep this in mind when creating your business cards.

Turn your invoice into a marketing tool

The humble invoice can be quite often overlooked as being nothing more than a record of a bill. But at the bottom of your invoice you can advertise a special offer or direct your customer to a special page on your website.

Alternatively, you can use the invoice to reaffirm your USP or seven reasons to buy again from you.

A special offer listed on the invoice might include a discount off a treatment or some other kind of incentive so that the person who has just received the treatment will go and share the benefits with some of their friends.

You might use the idea of referrals in exchange for a discount or free gift if the client actively refers new business your way.

As you may have already realised, direct referrals can have a huge impact on your business. The other good thing about an invoice is it that it has longevity.

If you are offering a treatment which can be used as a tax deduction for the client, whenever they do their books your little offer will be staring back at them.

It might be that they will receive 20% off their next treatment with a heading like:

"Claim your Tax Return Special Offer before the end of financial year"

or *"Tired of doing your Tax Return? Sounds like you need a massage. Book a treatment before June 30th and receive a 90 minutes massage for the price of a 1 hour massage".*

If your client is doing the books in preparation for the end of the tax year it might just be the thing they need. Also remember that any offer you make should always feature an expiry date.

Free reports

You may be asking yourself, what is a free report? A free report is an email information package which gives your clients an overview of the products or services you offer. Your free report should include a description of your services; a description of what your modality is; and, lists the benefits of the treatments.

Free reports also include testimonials from your existing clients and a special offer to entice your readers to take action. For example, a call to action might be: *"Make a booking within 7 days of receiving this email and receive a free gift valued at $20.00"*.

When it comes to free reports, your customers want information without the hassle of having to phone your business. Here the customer can read the information at their leisure.

I always arrange a PDF version of the free reports that I send out so that they can be easily emailed in addition to my other promotional emails. Alternatively, you can offer hard copies for those who prefer it. When crafted correctly, free reports work exceedingly well to motivate customers to do business with you.

E-newsletters

Email newsletters are an excellent way to keep in contact with your existing clientele and to keep them up-to-date with your latest offers. If you have not done so already you should be compiling a database of all your clients in a data file program such as *Excel*.

Be sure to gain your client's permission to send them email. If you have gained their permission, whenever you send your clients one of your e newsletters they will welcome them. Without permission, you are sending unsolicited email or *spam*.

An E-newsletter is one of the most cost effective ways to maintain contact with your clients and costs you nothing more than a little time and an internet connection. You can send out one email to your entire database or to specific target groups provided you have the right programs for bulk, yet personalised email.

Alternatively, you can send generic emails to your clients with a general headline in the subject heading but this approach can miss the mark and is sometimes ignored or captured as bulk email ending up on the recipient's spam folder.

You can avoid this by ensuring your emails are sent as *text*, rather than in *html* code with attached images in the email. Although html email format looks great, you have a higher strike rate over sending email in a text format. Most people have anti-spam software which targets *html* code, thus preventing your email being read.

When creating your e newsletter it is important that you keep the information interesting. There should always be some news as well as an article or two, even if you are not the one writing them as you can get other practitioners to contribute to your newsletter.

The idea is that your newsletter isn't just a bunch of advertising with offers, it should offer some genuinely interesting information related to your field which clients will find beneficial. Of course, you should make some offer to entice your clients to visit again but ultimately your newsletters are there to remind your clients that you still exist and this way they will remember to do business with you again and again.

Client testimonials

Testimonials truly speak volumes. If you can obtain these from professionals within your industry as well as from your existing clients, the more received the better. Testimonials need only be a few lines long, stating clearly how your client has benefited from your treatments.

To kick start your testimonial list, ask your previous clients. You will find that many will be happy to help you. This is even more so when asking them face-to-face at the end of the treatment. You can do this by asking them if they would mind writing a few words explaining what they got out of your session.

Be sure to ask them if you have their permission to use their testimonial *(provided it's a positive response)* in your future advertising. You might even wish to type up a testimonial form page with a tick box where they give their consent for use of their testimonial in your advertising materials.

Although you should encourage constructive criticism, a juicy testimonial is what you are after, so set the scene from the beginning. You will be surprised just how many people are willing to write you a complimentary report.

Testimonials can then be used on your business cards; throughout your website; in your brochures; at the end of your email signatures and the like to tell the world just how amazing you truly are.

Gift vouchers

Gift vouchers are another item which you should offer to your existing clientele. In my treatment room, I have a large display and sign offering gift vouchers.

Here's an example of how your gift voucher might read...

'This gift voucher entitles the bearer to a 1 hour treatment with (your name). Certified practitioner (of your association, or school you studied with, or membership affiliation you have gained to add to your credibility)'.

You will often find that by advertising your gift vouchers, especially before Christmas as a gift for the person who has everything, can bring in a great deal of new business.

When it comes to gift vouchers it is recommended to put an expiry date. Otherwise five years later the recipient may call you saying, 'my friend *(of whom by this time, you have no recollection)* bought me this gift voucher'.

In the meantime you may have moved your business or put up your prices several times. A reasonable time frame for expiry dates is one to six months.

Graphic design

When it comes to producing your flyers and business cards, unless you have the skills in desktop publishing and a background in graphic design I strongly suggest you employ the skills and creative talents of a graphic designer.

If you attempt to design and produce your own flyers, they will in more cases than not, look home-made and thus convey a non-professional message to your potential clients.

When selecting a graphic designer, it is not necessary to go direct to a big graphic design studio as the fees per hour can be higher than what you may charge. When you take into account the amount of time it can take to get your cards just right, you may find you have spent a great deal even before going to the printer.

One way to get around this is to look for a freelance graphic designer. Often graphic designers who have just completed their training will be looking for new jobs for their folio and will be happy to offer you a reduced rate just to add 'real jobs' to their folio. *(I know because I used to be one!)*

When arranging a quote for graphic design always arrange a written quote prior to commencing the project and get your graphic designer to sign on this agreed price. In this way, you can be sure that if you need to go overtime you will not suffer financially as a result. If the graphic designer is worth their salt, they will know how to quote for a fair price and this will often reflect a better quote than those found at big graphic design studios.

If, on the other hand, you have a big advertising budget and can afford a professional design studio the money spent can produce some amazing work. It is really a question of what is possible and how far your money needs to stretch.

As always, get more than one quote for the same job as prices will vary from one designer to another. When selecting your graphic designer you need to ensure they are of a suitable standard, so arrange a meeting to view their work or visit their website (if they have one) and check out their style and ability.

You may also wish to determine whether they have skills in website production because they will be able to translate the same design elements from your business card and flyers to a website with little difficulty.

In-house printing designers

Some printers now offer in-house graphic design. Although they usually charge fewer fees per hour than graphic design studios, they can often lack the creative flair of graphic designers. As with freelance, studio or in-house designers you need to do your homework to determine which designer is most suitable.

DIY desktop publishing

If you are looking to save money, then DIY Desktop Publishing may be an entry level option for creating your business cards and flyers. Many desktop publishing programs now offer ready made templates for business cards and flyers, where you simply insert your details and the template will automatically change the type face, and colours to suit your needs.

Many of these software programs offer diverse choices and you will have many options for choosing several different type faces and effects such as drop shadows, wacky fonts and clip art images for your flyers.

The principle motto is: *keep it simple.* For many, there is a tendency to put several type faces on the same card with every effect so as to make your card stand out. However, the result does stand out but not in a good way. You want to be remembered for how your card reflects your business not how impressive and diverse your desktop publishing program can be.

Another alternative is to take a short course on how to operate these publishing software programs. Many local schools offer after-hours training or you may wish to employ the private tuition of a graphic designer to teach you how to use them.

For more information on desktop publishing read the *'For Dummies'* series, such as *'Desktop Publishing for Dummies'*.

Getting ready for the printer

Once you have a design that you are happy with, be this via the graphic designer, in-house designer, or relying on your DIY desktop publishing ability, you will need to save the document in a format that your printer will be able to use. Failing to do this will result in additional time and untold irritation for both you and the printer.

If you have a graphic designer doing your job then they will have already sorted this out for you. Most printers these days accept the format of PDF for printing. In most design programs such as ILLUSTRATOR, COREL DRAW, QUARK and PAGEMAKER, you will have the option of saving your file as a High Resolution PDF. This file (providing it is not too big) can then be emailed to your printer ready for printing.

Once you have submitted your artwork for printing you will need to select the stock or paper for the print job. Here there are many choices as to whether to go with a standard paper or 100% recycled paper which is quite a bit more expensive but very environmental.

The paper you are printing on also needs to be taken into consideration with regards the colours you are using in the design process. Paper from printers is measured in weight or

GSM. There is also a big difference in weight or how flimsy or sturdy the paper is between gloss paper and non-gloss paper. Generally gloss is more flimsy when compared to non-gloss when rated at the same weight so one should take this into consideration when ordering paper.

If you visit the printer you are happy with they will be able to give you free samples of various papers and weights so take the time to consider the stock and price before making a decision.

Chapter 7

Advertising: Where and How

It makes sense that if you are going to advertise your natural therapy business you need to know where to advertise and how big your ad should be. In this chapter I will guide you through the world of advertising and detail which methods bring in the best results.

Where to advertise – Local or national?

The age old question of where to advertise depends on where you practice and how far you wish to travel (if at all), to share your professional services with others. If you want people to come to your premises or home for your treatments, there is not much point in advertising to potential clients who live hours away. Unless you're the greatest practitioner on earth, they are not likely to travel vast distances to receive a treatment from you.

If you offer mobile treatments on the other hand, and are prepared to travel to give treatments to others, you first need to determine how far you are willing to travel. Once you have established your distance, it makes little sense to advertise in publications beyond this boundary.

Your local community newspaper or magazine can be a great resource and one should not underestimate the benefits of these mediums for advertising.

For example at my clinic I advertise in the local paper and receive several calls for bookings from this small classified ad each week.

Knowing your target audience

The next thing you should consider is your target audience.

There is not much use in advertising in magazines which have nothing to do with your services. Just because a sales person contacts you because they have a great advertising offer does not mean you should see it as a sign from the heavens to spend your advertising budget on an audience who is not interested in your services.

It makes sense to research various magazine readerships and test these mediums before committing to a series of advertisements. Many advertising sales people will offer you great deals for advertising on the same ad over six issues or more but if your ad does not work the first time it will not work for the other issues either. Remember you need to check the results of all your advertising.

Yellow Pages advertising

In the *Yellow Pages* most natural therapies are listed under the category of Alternative Health Therapies and Services. You would be surprised just how little you need to spend on yellow pages advertising to stand out from the crowd.

For many therapists, I recommend advertising in such a way that asks your potential client to find out more.

Ideally your website or toll free number should be listed. Because it can be quite expensive to have even a small display advertisement in the *Yellow Pages*, you are much better off having a simple teaser listing where they will be compelled to find out more.

The following is a simple formula that brings results, of course you can tailor the advertisement specifically to your target audience but the fundamental elements remain the same.

Your name and business name in bold - *Qualified Therapist.*

Need energy? Guaranteed secret to restore vitality! Discover how, phone: (your phone number) or visit: www.yourwebsite.com for a free information kit valued at $37.00.

In this simple example, the bold heading with your name or business name will draw the reader to your listing. You may even consider the bold heading in a red spot colour. This will draw the reader's eye even more.

Let us now look at why this simple ad works.

The statement: *'Need energy? Guaranteed secret to restore vitality!'*.

This identifies your customer's problem and offers a solution to their problem. It also calls them to act with the statement: *'Discover how'*.

The statement: *'Qualified Therapist'* tells your future client that you have credibility and know what you are doing. It tells them you are qualified and that you are able to help them with their problems. With the statement: *'Guaranteed'* you are removing the element of risk by telling your potential client that they are assured a result by receiving your treatment. It also tells them that you are so sure of the effectiveness of your treatment you are willing to guarantee it.

Adding your phone number and website for a free information kit gives your potential client the opportunity to find out more information. The fact that they will receive a free report valued at $37.00 is reason enough to take action.

If you do not have a website, you can offer a Free Report via email. In this case, your last line can read as follows: *Discover how, email: yourname@serviceprovider.com for a free information kit valued at $37.00.*

As you can see every word counts and drives home a clear message and call to action. If you create your advertisement well you will be successful in flagging down new clients.

Press advertising

Press advertising is another powerful medium which need not cost the earth. Small space advertisements can really have a hypnotic effect on the reader. One of the best ways to have your ad read is to not make your ad look like an ad. If advertising is the very thing your reader is not interested in, why not make your ad look like an article? One way to achieve this is to produce an ad which looks like a newspaper article. This is where a strong headline does over 80% of the work for you.

The following are some proven attention grabbing headlines which work:

'10 steps to renewed health and vitality'
'Learn the secret to living without back pain'
'Discover the natural energy renewal technique everyone is talking about'
'Astonishing facts about natural healing you must read'
'You can heal yourself! Healing secrets revealed by local therapist'
'Secret healing technique aids cancer patient'
'Attention migraine sufferers! Astonishing health secret revealed'
'Do you have what it takes to live pain-free?'
'The truth about meditation, the secrets revealed'
'7 healing secrets everyone should know'

Once you have flagged down your reader's interest, you can go on to reveal your important <u>must read</u> message. Your article also known as 'advertorial' can then be written in such as way which highlights the key benefits. You may also wish to write your article in an interview format. Whichever way you choose, because your ad is no longer looking like an ad you will have a far higher chance of being read.

The power of classified ads
A classified advertisement is not only a tool to revealing why someone should use your service, it is designed to elicit interest and entice the reader to find out more. In a classified ad you do not have enough space to tell your story. You have only a few

lines to grab the reader's attention and establish a call to action.

Just in the same way that the previous headlines offered some powerful statements which grab the reader's interest, the same headlines can be used in classified ads with similar effect.

Here are some examples:

Free report reveals: The 10 steps to health and happiness. *Email:* *info@serviceprovider.com to find out how or call: (your phone number).*

Introductory offer – Free Bowen treatment from qualified therapist *(Offer expires June 30th). Limited to the first 15 callers only. Ring Now! Ph: (your phone number).*

No energy? *Don't miss your chance to experience Reiki today. Proven results from (your city's) leading therapist. Phone: (your phone number).*

Ideally your classified ad should be no more than 30 words and ideally less. Because there are so many classified ads in most health and new age publications you need an attention grabbing headline or statement to flag down the reader. When writing your classified ads the most important thing to remember is a strong headline. Unless your headline arrests the reader the rest of your ad doesn't matter because no one will read it.

Magazine advertising

Magazine advertising like press can be very expensive, but unlike newspaper advertising where the readership is general, with magazines you can choose your target audience more specifically. There are many publications on the market these days on the subjects of health, spirituality and personal growth. Just in the same way that it is not necessary to advertise a full page, small space advertising, if done effectively, can do wonders for your business.

Radio advertising and talk-back-interviews

Radio is an all too often overlooked medium which can bring tremendous results. This is not necessarily in the form of the usual ads you get on commercial radio, because just like press and magazine advertising where ads that look like ads are largely ignored, so it is with radio. Most radio ads sound like radio ads and people tend to tune out or switch stations.

People listen to the radio for music, the announcers and interviews. Herein lays one of the best forms of radio advertising. You would be surprised just how many calls you will receive by being interviewed on the radio about your natural therapy.

The best way to achieve this is to call several radio stations (not just the large commercial ones) to see which stations have segments dedicated to Mind, Body, Spirit, or Health. Talk back radio segments are ideal and if you only have one minute air time or even a brief mention, it can still be enormously beneficial for your business.

To give you an example, some years ago one of our local and very well known radio celebrities attended our weekly Reiki clinic. He headed up a popular morning talkback show and used some of his experiences as raw materials for his daily shows.

Although the content had a 'tongue in cheek' feel the exposure was great. As a result the station received dozens of calls from people wanting to find out more about Reiki. Subsequently, our clinic (which was running at a modest pace), suddenly became booked out for weeks in advance.

When your natural therapy receives a good endorsement from a high profile celebrity, the benefits are far reaching. Publicity for your modality whether it is in the form of a radio interview, magazine article or other media not only benefits your practice but everyone else in your profession.

Television advertising

Television is another great medium for free exposure. One way to get free exposure is to target lifestyle programs. In particular, programs which are dedicated to health, lifestyle, or wellness. You may even get a chance to appear on travel programs if the program is looking at things to do when they feature your town.

Simply pick up a copy of the local television guide and see which programs your services may fall into. All you need to do is call the television stations and see if they are interested in doing a segment on your natural therapy. Of course, you will get plenty of knock backs but you have nothing to lose and if you receive only one 'yes' that is all you need.

Another alternative is to fax a press release to the television stations. Give the station an overview of what you offer and how this may be of interest to their audience.

Lifestyle programs which are scheduled for prime time viewing are also worthy of consideration. You don't want to be on television at 3am, along with the shopping channels so it is best to try for breakfast shows or early evening programs ideally scheduled between 5pm and 9pm.

Direct point of sale

In addition to your usual means of promotion it may also be worth considering other direct ways to promote your business. These include: Bumper Stickers; Fridge Magnets; Car Magnets; Postcards; and, Book Marks. It can be relatively inexpensive to produce these additional tools for promotion. Let us now take a look at these one by one.

Bumper stickers

Compared to the price of a business card, a bumper sticker can be more costly, especially if you are choosing to go the whole way and produce full-colour stickers which are UV protected for outdoor use, but a bumper sticker makes your business mobile and has greater longevity than a business card. The idea with a bumper sticker is that you want people to read it. Try to engage your reader with something that draws attention to the bumper sticker which is also memorable and relevant to your business.

Fridge magnets

Another relatively inexpensive alternative are fridge magnets. The humble fridge magnet serves a function that business cards can not and that is that they live on the fridge door and are seen daily. The other added benefit is that people tend to keep fridge magnets not just for a day or week but sometimes for years.

Of course there is no point in ordering 1000 fridge magnets if nobody has them. You need to find creative ways to get your magnets out to new as well as your existing customers.

The first thing you can do is implement a mail-out to all of your existing customers. Send two fridge magnets and two 50% off gift vouchers for your next treatment.

Your cover letter might read as follows: *"Please stick this magnet on your fridge as you will need it to hold the enclosed gift vouchers for 50% of your next consultation"*. Then ask your customer to give one of these fridge magnets to a friend along with one of your gift vouchers. Remind them that your business is all about personal service and sharing what you do via word of mouth. If you ask customers to refer on, they often will.

Another way to get your fridge magnets on other fridges is to contact fellow practitioners and ask them if they will be willing to do some cross promotion.

You can take some of their business cards or flyers and put them in your clinic in exchange for having some of your flyers; business cards, magnets etc, displayed in their clinic.

The idea is that as you cross-refer you generate new business from each other's clientele. When anyone makes enquiries and would like some further information about your practice be sure to put at least two or three fridge magnets and business cards in with your information pack.

Another application for the humble fridge magnet is to turn

your fridge magnet into a yearly calendar. It only needs to be business card size (90mm x 55mm) listing the months and dates. At the bottom of the pocket calendar you feature your USP and contact details. In this way you create advertising for your business that also serves a practical purpose.

Car magnets

Why not use your car as a magnet for your business. Most business owners drive a car on a daily basis. Having a car magnet is truly mobile advertising. Car magnets are cost-effective and give your business added exposure. In addition to placing the car magnets on either side of your car you may also choose to list your website on the rear window or bumper.

When you think about how many cars drive behind you, it makes sense that you have every opportunity to promote your business to the unsuspecting traveler.

Instead of putting something really boring like your name and phone number, why not use an engaging catchphrase with your phone number and website.

For example: *"Don't just sit there, you can feel better now the natural way!" Call Fremantle Naturopathy Clinic on 9335 1133. Your first consultation is free!*

Because most mobile phones have built-in cameras these days, many people will either type in your phone number or visit your website using their mobile phone. They might even take a photo of your details with their mobile for future reference.

If you are going to go for the car magnets mobile advertisement, remember to keep your message short, distinct, relevant and memorable. Like most forms of advertising you only have about one second to flag down the driver's interest, unless they are stuck behind you in traffic!

The last thing to consider is the quality of your vehicle. If your car is due to breakdown any minute and looks like it has been in a demolition car race then this may not be the most suitable vehicle to draw attention to. Most people will think that you are not very successful if you drive a shabby looking car. Although some people may take pity on you it will not display a positive first impression.

This is not to say that you need to get a brand new car, but it might be worth spending a little bit more in order to gain a good first impression if you are using your car to promote your business. I have a few friends who choose the colour of their new car based on the colours of their business logo. Is that going too far? I don't think so.

Expos, psychic fairs and competitions

These days there are a variety of expos for mind, body and spirit. These events are a prime opportunity to promote your natural therapy practice. If you intend to participate in an expo and obtain a stall to offer treatments you will need to consider just how many new clients you will need to obtain in order to cover your expenses.

An alternative way to offset the costs is to share your stall with a fellow practitioner or join a group of practitioners from a health spa or healing group to reduce your expenses.

To ensure you cover your costs and generate new clients, it is essential to give expo visitors a special offer to secure future bookings. You might also wish to run a competition. An example might be where expo visitors fill out a coupon to be in the running to win a series of free treatments or some other prize of your choice.

In the meantime, you will have obtained numerous phone numbers, addresses and emails to notify all those who did not win with a follow-up special offer. For example, you might write a letter or send an email along the following lines:

Dear (insert person's first name),

I am writing this email to thank you for participating in our 'win 3 free treatments competition' featured at the recent Mind Body Spirit expo. Unfortunately, your name was not drawn for the major prize however, as a consolation I would like to offer you a 'Buy one, get one free trial offer'. If you make a booking before (date of your choosing) you can take advantage of this 'not to be missed' special offer. Simply phone....to make a booking.

Please also find enclosed some information about (your practice) as well as some testimonials from previous clients who benefited from my services.

I look forward to hearing from you at your nearest opportunity.

Signed, (your name, position and business name).

PS. You can also visit: (insert your website address) to be in the running for our next competition.

Running a competition and sending out letters or emails in this manner can really add new clients to your practice plus the participants will also appreciate being offered a consolation prize.

Me mail, not email

When it comes to email I recommend you make all your emails personalised. Use the person's first name when sending email as opposed to sending email with: *'Dear customer'*. If you do not personalise your email, the person will simply delete your email along with all the other spam in their inbox.

It is also essential to choose very carefully the subject heading for your emails, especially if you are making contact with a new email recipient for the very first time.

Unlike standard special offers where you offer something free or offer a discount, if you type these headlines into a subject heading most people will also read these as spam and delete the email.

To ensure email readership, I usually type in the recipient's name with the words: *For (person's name) from (listing your name or business name).* This ensures higher readership and does not look like advertising email even though this is what you may be offering.

When making a special offer make sure you are making an offer to someone who is looking for such an offer and that you have their permission to send them an email. It needs to be relevant to the customer.

I usually achieve this in a two-step fashion. I first call the person and ask them if they would be willing to receive some further information about our services and a special offer for their consideration. Provided I receive their permission to send them an email, I make sure the email is received by the right person in the right department. I also advise the person of the title of the subject heading and when they should expect to receive the email. This process does take a great deal longer but the time spent will be well worth it.

Nobody wants to be offered some thing which is not relevant to them. For example, if you walked into a hardware store and someone came up to you an offered you a great travel deal, you would probably just switch off. You are shopping for hardware items and you don't want to be offered something which as nothing to do with your purpose for shopping. Likewise make your offers relevant to your customers and your hit rate will be far higher.

Up-selling verses discounting
Most therapists think that the best way to get new clients is to offer a discount but what this means is that you will get less money for working the same amount of time. In order to land new clients a discount like 50% off your first consultation can be

a great way to attract new clients, even a free introductory treatment works wonders but you should only discount in the beginning. Once you have won them over to continue to discount only means you get less money for your time. It's a false economy and will leave you working more hours with less reward.

The best thing to do once you have secured new clients is to up-sell. What this means is to entice your clients to buy again by giving them something extra. This is where you offer a package treatment or a series.

I'll give you a recent example from a fellow practitioner who was requesting some advice on his new practice. He started out giving a 1 hour massage treatment at half price at the opening of his clinic. This worked wonders because he got loads of new clients who were really happy to give him a try because it was a really good deal.

His offer also had a time limit. It expired within a few weeks. This was a good idea as it presented a clear call to action in order to receive the 50% discount.

After the special had run its course the time came for a new offer. He suggested to me that he would offer the same treatments to the same clients, this time at 30% off. Big mistake! His existing clients would feel a little disappointed that they had to pay more for the same thing, even if it was discounted in the first place. I suggested he change the deal and offer an up-sell. Instead of discounting, I suggested the up-sell of a treatment package. The up-sell read like this.

"Book three treatments before (expiry date) and your fourth treatment is free.

Save $75.00! – Offer closes February 30th. Book now to reserve your place."

On the advertisement the special also read: *Four treatments are normally: $300. Book today and pay only: $225. Save $75.00!*

Who doesn't want to save $75.00? The thing is people focus on what they save and do not think about the money they have invested. Now instead of getting less, he secured an additional two treatments which he may not have previously had on the old system. The added bonus is that his clients paid in advance.

Treatments booked in advance means money in the bank. You don't have the problem of people canceling or just not showing up. Nothing guarantees attendance at a session more than payment in advance. The rule of thumb is you need to re-think your current offers and keep them fresh to entice your clients to buy again and again.

Coupon lines

Would you like to know how to increase the readership of your advertisements by up to 500%? What if I told you that you could achieve this by a series of small lines?

The answer is simple, all you do is add coupon cut out lines around your advertisements and classifieds. For example:

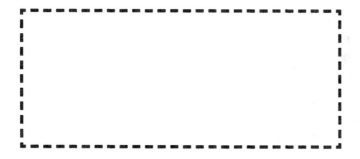

Coupon cut out lines increase readership dramatically. Over the years our brains are simply conditioned to identify coupon outlines as it is a symbol associated with a special offer. This works particularly well for newspaper advertising or classifieds where your advertisement is competing with other headlines and lots of dominate black and white. Be sure to utilise this in part or on all of your advertising in conjunction with an attention grabbing headline.

A spot of colour

Adding a spot colour (in particular the colour red) adds an equally arresting quality to press advertising. This is even more so when your advertisement or classified ad is the only one listed in the colour red. The eye naturally goes to the colour.

If you are planning on advertising in a newspaper type publication, first check a previous issue. If no previous advertiser is using spot colour, make enquiries to see if you will be able to add a spot colour for an additional rate. Your chances of being read first are assured.

It may cost you as much as double as the cost of the original black and white ad but it will be money well spent. Listing your headline in bold and in red type will attract readership dramatically.

Add or remove the .00's

If you are offering a discount or an added value to your service, add the decimal points. The reason for this is that it makes the amount appear to be a higher value.

For example: *First 30 callers receive a free gift valued at $30.00.*

If we leave off the .00's the offer reads: *First 30 callers receive a free gift valued at $30.*

Alternatively when you are advertising the price that you are charging for your services always remove the decimal point. For example: *Secure your investment now for only $47.* When you remove the decimal point for an amount to be paid it looks like it costs less.

Positive and negative money words

When listing your fee associated with the offer, do not use negative money words such as *fee* or *cost.* Instead use positive

money words such as *investment* or *value*. For example:
   'All this for the added value of $95.00!' or *'your investment is only $147'.*

Say it with an exclamation mark!

Adding an exclamation mark at the end of a headline or special offer makes your statement stand out. It also makes the statement appear more exciting. What is being read in the reader's mind is being shouted and has a sense of urgency.

For example: *Save $527.00 this month!* If it is really big news, add three exclamation marks. *Save $527.00 this month!!!*

Prices that work

I don't know why this is the case but when you advertise services with the numbers ending with 7 and 9, the success rates are higher. The following prices work particularly well: $27; $37; $47; $97; $127; $147; $247; $379 and so on. Remember to remove the decimal points when advertising the price and add words like: only; just; introductory; offer; special, as these words make the price even more appealing.

Chapter 8

The Secret of Permission Marketing

In this chapter I will share with you one of the most effective ways to reach new customers who will actually anticipate and welcome your marketing messages. Sounds hard to believe? Read on.

When it comes to marketing there are essentially two kinds. There is the kind you ignore, the other you adore. The first and most long-standing kind is called interruption marketing. Interruption marketing as the name suggests, is where the marketing interrupts your life. This can take many forms such as the advertisements that come on in the middle of a television program. It also includes the advertising you hear on commercial radio, as well as the advertisements you see everywhere such as the ones listed in the newspaper, on billboards, and in junk mail. The list is endless.

Interruption marketing is everywhere and has and still dominates the marketplace. Today the marketplace is saturated with so much advertising. All of the advertisers are competing for your attention. You only have to walk down the street or watch 30 minutes of television and you will be bombarded with what appears to be endless advertising messages. The same applies online. Go to most websites and you will usually come across some form of banner advertising or a flash feature designed to grab your attention.

We are also all familiar with the endless multitude of spam email, which seems to be ever increasing. No matter what we try, be it the latest anti-spam software applications, still more spam rears its ugly head.

Now if we go back 20 years the amount of advertising many people were exposed to was considerably less. People watched less television, the internet was not commonplace, and you could go to a public toilet and not have a poster looking back at you. Back then we also probably responded to more of this advertising simply because there was less of it.

But these days we are getting busier and busier and have less time to take in more messages than ever before. Therefore, advertisers and marketers have to try even harder to catch our attention. It becomes a never-ending cycle. Because we are very busy as consumers and have less time to notice the greater amounts of advertising, the advertisers increase the advertising so that we take notice of them. This only makes consumers feel even more overwhelmed and we unconsciously block out more and more of the endless advertising messages.

So how do we break into the consumer's mind using *the Secrets of Spiritual Marketing?* We do so with their expressed permission.

Let me run a scenario for you. Let's suppose that you are shopping in the supermarket and a friend of yours comes up to you and says: *"Hi Bob, how are you going?"*.

In the course of the conversation your friend mentions that he has just tried a new product. He speaks about how he had enjoyed it, how he found it to be really useful and recommends the product to you. Then it just so happens that right there where you are standing the product is on display. Listed on the product are all of the benefits written in a clear and straightforward manner. There isn't too much information listed on the product which is a good thing as you have little time and are busy shopping at the supermarket, so you buy the product on the spot.

Do you think you would be likely to buy the product after hearing your trusted friend's report? The answer, of course, is most likely.

However, if you were shopping and glanced at the product, if it caught your eye in the first place, chances are you would not buy this product.

This illustrates the difference between permission and interruption. In this little scenario your friend has given you information and you listen because it comes from a trusted source. No hard sell plus no motive to sell on behalf of your friend.

When we hear about something with permission we are more likely to buy than without permission.

Interruption marketing, on the other hand, robs you of your time. Interruption marketing is a little bit like a thief. There you are walking down the street, minding your own business and interruption marketing stops you to steal some of your time. If the message isn't relevant or engaging do you think you will be inclined to buy the item or service? The end result is that the consumer and the advertiser both lose.

Permission marketing, on the other hand, does the exact opposite. It is marketing which is welcomed. It is relevant and can even be anticipated by the consumer because the consumer has volunteered to receive it. Unlike interruption marketing, permission marketing enables you to have an attentive audience who actually wants to receive the information you are presenting because it is of interest to them. Unfortunately, in order to create this relationship, all permission marketing and advertising requires some initial interruption marketing to start the relationship unless it begins via word of mouth.

The trick is to create an avenue where the consumer will volunteer to be involved with what you are offering and one needs to cultivate this relationship stage by stage. For example, you may offer some kind of incentive such as joining an online newsletter for the latest updates and information about your product and service. Because you have done your homework and identified the customers who want this information, they have opted in to receive your email newsletters.

In this way you have gained their interest either through interruption marketing where you advertised in a specialist magazine or by direct mail order, or telemarketing to achieve this result.

By slowly growing the business relationship you build their confidence and trust in the service you are offering. By building this relationship you can gradually build sales. Once you build sales you reward your customers with excellent service because you have recognised the lifetime value of your customer.

Permission marketing also takes the form of referral advertising through friends who are using the same product or service. It also can take the form through networks such as *forums* where friends introduce their friends to a product or service but without all of the hype and hard sell that most people have a clear aversion to.

The various levels of permission

In Seth Godin's book *'Permission Marketing'* he writes about 5 levels of Permission.

These are:

1. Intravenous
2. Points
3. Personal relationships
4. Brand trust
5. Situation

Rather than spelling out all of these in great detail what follows is a brief summary in relation to practitioners in the wellness industry.

Intravenous

The first and highest level of permission is 'Intravenous'. In a nutshell this means the customer has given you permission to make their buying decisions for them. For example, your client may buy a regular product from you on a monthly basis or come for weekly treatments. Through a complete stroke of luck the client has said to you:

"Look, I keep coming here weekly, here's my credit card number, just debit my account each week".

This is what you call the dream client or the Direct Debit Client.

A great many big business operations are set up in this way and you too can make this kind of offer to your regular clients. Whether weekly or monthly, this is by far the best level of permission.

Points

The second level of permission is 'Points'. A point system is where the customer collects points each time they use a product or service. Think airline frequent flyer programs; your local coffee shop loyalty card where your 10th cup is free, or, a discount off your petrol when you collect your shopper dockets.

A points system promotes customers to buy again. As a natural therapist, you could have a loyalty card where your 5th treatment is free or you qualify for a special discount after a certain number of treatments.

I know that I go out of my way to collect points with my credit card and a points system can be a great way to retain customers and encourage them to use and re-use your products and services.

Personal relationships

The third level of permission is 'Personal relationships'. This is where you build relationships with your existing clients. It is far easier to share a new product with a friend than with a stranger going in cold. If you are a natural therapist you have a unique opportunity to build relationships with your clients. After all you do meet them in person.

There are many things you can do to build the client relationship. Some of the best ways is to remember their name, their birthday or give them a gift out of the blue. Remember your last conversation and ask them about themselves outside the treatments.

The point is not to cross the line and start going out on lunch dates or to the movies, but you can still maintain the professional relationship and build it on a personal level at the same time.

Once you have a customer's trust the next step is the intravenous level, where you become trustworthy and are seen not only as *a therapist*, you become *their therapist*. There is a big difference with this transition. This is where they become a client for life. This level also ensures your client will refer their friends and give testimonials, especially if you ask them to.

Brand Trust

'Brand Trust' is the fourth level of permission. Your brand in this case is you. In other cases it is your business name or the unique service or treatment you offer. This is all wrapped up in your USP – Unique Selling Proposition.

Brand trust is largely out there because of a great deal of repetition. Think Volvo for safety, Coke for soft drinks or Starbucks for coffee. The trust is there because it has a long track record.

This level applies to you the longer you are in practice and the more you position your USP in the marketplace.

The Reiki Institute* I founded is well known because of years of advertising and web presence. We established a professional standard which today is recognised with quality and service. The longer someone is familiar with your product and service as well as your name, the greater the brand trust engendered.

*See: www.reikitraining.com.au

Situation

The last level of permission marketing is 'Situation'. This is where the customer is in direct contact and asking you for more information.

A good example is when someone calls your toll free number and asks to book a treatment or they would like some more information. They have sought you out and you have an opportunity to sell and then up-sell. Think: 'Would you like fries with that?'. How could you get your customers to upgrade their order when calling you? Perhaps it's a treatment package or series booking. If you don't ask you could be knocking back more business without knowing it.

A warning about the business relationship

Never and I mean NEVER take advantage of your business relationship. If you have attained the 'holy grail' in permission where your client has given you authorisation to auto renew or direct debit their credit card for your services, never abuse this level of permission by over-charging their credit card or breaching your client's privacy by sharing their sensitive information with other parties. No sooner than any breach of the client's trust occurs, then you'll find your client is no longer a client.

Another thing you should never do is force a sale with 'marketing threats'. Now you may be thinking who would do such a thing and what is a 'marketing threat'?, I'll give you an example. Some months ago I responded to an offer to receive a free newsletter on marketing tips for natural therapists and being a keen researcher on such matters I happily subscribed to the free three-month newsletter which was advertised as being 'obligation free' and 'no strings attached'. The funny thing was that they requested my credit card number should I wish to upgrade to the newsletter's full package.

After receiving the three free e-newsletters I was sent a letter from the same marketing company warning me that unless I canceled my membership by making a call or sending them a fax (at my expense mind you – no toll free number) that they would automatically charge my credit card $49.97 every month until the end of time. Their offer had the words WARNING in big bold letters and a threat that

"... *You must be completely satisfied. If not, I want you to cancel your membership*". They want me to cancel my membership?

From someone who should know better, they immediately lost a customer for life, my confidence in their services and especially my trust.

I also made a point of educating them on exactly what they have done in terms of breaching my trust. I consider this approach to be very stupid.

After all, the money they had invested in wooing me for three months with free newsletters, they lost a client faster than they had acquired one. Permission means exactly this, you have the customer's permission, so never break it and you will enjoy the benefits of a long and prosperous business relationship.

Chapter 9

Advertising Myths and Mistakes

In this chapter I will illustrate some of the common myths and mistakes advertisers make. If you are like most natural therapists, you work hard to make a living and you want to make every advertising dollar work to bring you in new and renewed business.

The following myths break many rules most advertisers swear by, which is probably why most ads fail.

Advertising is one of those things that you can spend an awful lot of money on with little or no response, especially if you fail to follow proven strategies for success. The tragedy is that many practitioners have no idea how to advertise themselves and continue to advertise every week, or monthly for years, hoping that just having their name in the marketplace will eventually bring in new clientele. Unfortunately for the most part, this waiting game can land you with empty pockets in no time at all.

The good news is that in this chapter you will find indispensable tools which will not only save you hundreds of dollars but will dramatically increase clients.

Before I illustrate how to create advertising that generates enquiries and bookings, let's look at some of the more common myths about advertising you should avoid.

Myth #1
Bigger is better
Although a bigger ad will often draw more attention, it may not translate into business unless you know how to sell yourself. Over the years I have seen that small space ads can be just as effective, if not more than one big advertisement. Bigger is not

always favourable and if you are advertising in press or magazine publications, you can spend a lot of money for little results. Of course, advertisers will tell you that a bigger ad will generate more sales, but that is what they are trained to tell you. To sell more advertising space is the main aim of magazines and newspapers.

Myth #2
Repetition increases response

Another common advertising myth is that of repetition. Many sales people will tell you that it is enough to keep putting your name out there month after month, year after year, as eventually people will notice your advertising. For the most part they will notice your advertising but will not necessarily act upon it.

The fact of the matter is not how many times your advertisement is repeated but the content of the advertising which counts.

One ad can generate hundreds of calls over another, depending upon the content. You have to check what you are saying and if it is not working, you need to change it.

Holding out on the thought that by the third or fourth month, people will see your ad is costly yet so many people do this month after month.

We should have the philosophy that every dollar spent on advertising, marketing and promoting your business should always translate into more dollars for your business than the initial expense. If your advertising and marketing is not doing this, then this is what is called 'running your business at a loss'.

Myth #3
Ads should look like ads

Another common myth is that your ad should look like other ads. When I read a magazine, I want to read the magazine for its articles. I don't buy a magazine to read the ads. When you create your ad to look like an article in the magazine, you will guarantee higher readership and ultimately greater sales. This includes attention grabbing headlines to flag down the reader.

Myth #4
Cosmetic ads sell

Another common advertising myth is that your ad's appearance should look cosmetic or fancy. The use of full colour, high definition artistic photography and little copy may work for Coke or Sony but you aren't a global corporation with decades of product branding to be instantly recognised. It can be the case that when your ad looks too polished, people will simply gloss over it, thinking that whatever you are offering must be too expensive.

Myth #5
Too much copy drops readership

Another advertising myth is that if you put too much information into an advertisement, no one will read the copy.

The truth of the matter is that nothing could be further from the truth.

In fact, the more you tell, the more you sell.

Even if you are doing a small classified ad that only costs you a small fee every month, you can offer your readers access to information via your website or offer them a free information pack in the mail.

Your future clients want to know 'what's in it for them', so your free information kit is a way to persuade them to use your service. If you have the budget for a larger ad, then use all the available space to tell your story and give your reader every reason to buy.

How to create winning ads

The secret to creating winning ads is to produce ads that offer solutions to people's problems. The first thing you need to determine is, 'why would someone want to see you for treatments?'.

One simple way to find this out is to ask. Ask people you know who have received a treatment from you in the past and ask people who have not.

This is also a great way to renew old clients as well as generating new clients who may be interested by trying a session. The idea of a survey is to ask at least 50 people, and ideally 100 or more. Think of the level of business you will drum up just by doing this exercise.

Offer solutions to problems

Having conducted this exercise, you might find that some of the more common responses to the question include:

- Feeling out of balance.
- Feeling tired.
- Emotionally drained or going through emotional problems.
- To heal a specific injury or various aches and pains.

These are but a few of the common responses you will encounter. Now you need to wrap these reasons into a definitive statement which provides a solution to their problems.

Perhaps you have already identified this through establishing your USP.

When you identify the solution to your client's problems they will be happy to do business with you because you can offer them a solution to make their life better.

Words to use

The words you choose for your advertising have a large impact on the results. From an early age we identify with words and the images these create. It is not so much the words but the emotions and images that words bring which motivate us towards pleasure or pain.

When you use the right words in your advertising headlines and copy you create positive images in the minds of your readers.

The following are words to use which are engaging and bring about positive emotions in the minds of people:

- free
- easy
- at last!
- truth
- guarantee
- results
- proven
- introducing
- announcing
- astonishing
- safe
- save money
- breakthrough
- how to
- unique opportunity
- you/your
- exclusive
- discover
- revolutionary
- health
- love
- new
- facts
- improved
- fantastic
- value
- revealing
- powerful
- free gift
- buy one, get one free
- 50% off
- half price

Words that sell

The following words are strong words that sell:

- comfort
- deserve
- happy
- fun
- instant
- now

- person's name
- you've won!
- profit
- proud
- trust
- benefit

Words to avoid

The following words are to be avoided where possible as they create negative emotions and images in the minds of people.

- bad
- contract
- cost
- deal
- death
- difficult
- failure
- hurt
- liability
- loss
- lose
- obligation
- pay
- price
- sign
- maybe
- hard
- decline

The following are examples of headlines which incorporate motivating words for your advertising.

For health products:

"Discover the new, safe, and proven way to enjoy renewed health and vitality. Results are guaranteed or it's free! How?
Visit: www.vitalityunlimited.com for details."

For Thought Field Therapy:

"Breakthrough to success! Revolutionary 30 second technique brings lasting results in love, finances and relationships. Tap your way to a happier life! Visit: www.tappingyourmind.com."

For Chinese massage:

"Free report reveals the astonishing truth about Chinese massage and how you can be pain free without medicines.
Email: freereport@chinesemassage.com to find out how."

For weight loss consultants:

"Announcing a revolutionary weight loss program taking the world by storm. Do you know the secret? Find out now, visit: www.yourideal-weight.com."

The call to action

Creating a deadline for your advertising creates urgency. This is a powerfully motivating factor when you want your customers to take action. We all know how it is when we have all the time in the world to do something. Time goes by and the next thing we know, we have forgotten all about it.

When you call people to action with an enticing offer like: *"Half price treatments are limited to the first 10 callers"* you will be surprised just how quickly the phone rings.

When you tell your client to act in more cases than not, they do.

An example which calls your client to action might be:

"Call before March 24th to receive your free gift valued at $47.00, no questions asked".

Your limited offer which is valid for the next 7 days may be in reality be your on-going offer, but for someone who sees your advertisement or classified ad for the first time, it is an opportunity not to be missed.

Of course, you need to keep your offers fresh and to change them regularly, so as not to seem like your 'one week only' special offer is actually every week (even though this might be the case). The idea is to mix things up and to keep your offers fresh for new and old readers too.

Offer a money back guarantee

Money back guarantees are one of the most effective strategies to guarantee sales, plus they add tremendous credibility to your product or service.

Look through any alternative or complimentary therapy magazine and you'll see an almost non-existent display of money back guarantees or any guarantees that matter. When you offer a guarantee it dissolves the risk associated with the buying decision. These days the trend is to offer not just the money back but money back plus 10%. This is, for the customer, a 'customer wins, you lose' principle.

When you think about how many people will actually ask for their money back over the amount of new business a 'money back plus 10% guarantee' brings in, the 10% risk to your business is covered with the amount of new clients who will buy because of your guarantee.

If you dissolve the risk by offering a rock solid guarantee you will generate a great deal more business as a direct result. When someone is making a purchase somewhere in the back of their mind is the thought, 'what if this does not work?'. If you offer a guarantee this thought instantly goes away.

Tracking your advertising results

With any form of advertising it is vitally important that you test your ads on a regular basis. If your ad seems to be working and you decide to book an advertising series in a magazine, be sure that you have the option in the booking contract to make changes to the ad before each new issue.

If you place an ad and you do not get a response, change your ad as soon as possible, unless you have money to burn. It is important to monitor your enquiries and if you have received none then change what you are doing immediately.

When you do receive calls, especially if you have advertised in more than one place, always ask the person where they saw your ad or how they heard about you. This way you will know which ad worked and which medium drew the most enquiries. Keep a tally of the number of calls made and from where. Also tally email enquiries or enquiries made from referrals or word of mouth. Within a short period of time you will be able to track which format is most effective for your business.

Once you have found a form of advertising that works, and continues to work, keep on doing the same thing until you notice a dramatic change. Not all advertising works well forever so continual monitoring is essential to the success of your business.

Most natural therapists will tell you that they want more clients and they address this by running more ads (usually not ones that work) in more publications. What this means is that they end up spending a great deal of money across many areas with little results.

Imagine you were shopping online and ordered a new product every month but it never arrived. Instead of bothering to check why it had not arrived you kept on re-purchasing the same product every month in the hope that one of these products would finally arrive. Months pass so you decide to try other online shop and begin purchasing the same product from other retailers. It sounds crazy doesn't it? Would you do this in real life? Of course you'd say no. But the point I am making is that most natural therapists do exactly this same thing month after month, year after year or until they go out of business.

Not tracking your advertising to see if it works is like purchasing the same product (ad space) monthly and not asking why it has not arrived. I always suggest you try to get one ad right and then extend your advertising net to other publications. Getting one ad right can often translate into having more clients than you can handle.

Take all the guess work out of your advertising by establishing a database in a spreadsheet program, such as *Excel,* and have this on your computer desktop so you can enter in the results of your advertising responses.

On most web forms for online bookings through your website you should include a number of buttons which ask the question *'Where did you hear about us?'*.

Every time you get a response online add this to your database.

In addition to keeping track of enquiries on your computer, you may also wish to keep an eye on your telephone enquiries. Each time a person makes an enquiry ask them where they heard about you and using a note pad and pen simply place a tick next to the appropriate advertising medium. At the end of each week you can tally the enquiries on your computer to track results.

Another recommendation I have is to keep an eye out for all advertising which flags down your interest particularly in the area of natural therapies. Each time you see an advertisement you like, tear it and file it for future reference and inspiration. Advertisements that work are an excellent source of inspiration for your own advertising in the future.

Hopefully by reading this book you will be more readily able to identify which ads work and which ads do not work.

Unfortunately, you will find that there will be more ads that do not work versus those that do.

The good news is that if you continually monitor all of your advertising and marketing efforts you will experience a huge increase in your results, plus you will save money because you won't be wasting your time on advertising which does not yield results.

How to write a great headline

In order to write a great headline you need to express what you want to say which provokes an engaging and emotional response. If you can appeal to the reader's ego (instead of your own) then you will strike a chord with your reader and give them a reason to read on. The trick to good headlines is getting inside your client's head. It has to be all about them and not about you.

Your headline needs to stop your reader dead in their tracks. If you are advertising in a magazine or newspaper you are competing with hundreds of ads, so how can you stand out from this ocean of paper and ink?

The following headline approaches work wonders:

Identify your audience
Attention migraine sufferers
Back pain?
Workaholics!
Single Mums

How to's and how they work for you
How to reduce stress and be happy
How to make more money in the wellness industry
How to be pain free in 30 days

Make it free
Free report reveals....

Free consultation to the first 30 callers

Free $30.00 gift when you make a booking by (insert date)

Ask a question

Do you suffer from allergies?

Do you smoke cigarettes?

What are seven secrets to deeper relaxation?

What treatment is best for your back?

Wanted!

Wanted – Volunteers for free beauty consultation

Wanted – Sore feet for reflexology trial

Wanted – Smokers for free health test

Focus on the guarantee

Guaranteed better sleep or your money back

Guaranteed results! New touch therapy reveals...

Guaranteed weight loss in 60 days or it's free

Warning!

Warning to all women, new report reveals.....

A warning all parents should read....

Warning: Are your medications killing you?

It's all about me

I never thought I could see without glasses until...

I couldn't believe it but I was pain free for the first time in years.

They all laughed when I said I would be a healer but now....

Give me some reasons

Three reasons why you cannot afford to...

Seven reasons to call me now

Five good reasons to switch to natural therapies

State your offer

30 day free trial or it's free

Grand opening special - 50% off

Free herbal treatment for the first 30 callers

Why?

Why more people book treatments here than anywhere else

Why our therapists come to you

Why we give you more for your money

Make news!

Breakthrough formula to help you shed 10 kilos in 3 weeks!

At last! A revolutionary new way to cure snoring!

The secret weight-loss technique without counting kilos!

Take the challenge

Take this health quiz. Are you secretly unwell?

Take the 30 day liver cleansing challenge!

Are you qualified to massage your baby?

These are just a few angles you can take to dramatically improve your headlines and increase your readership.

Above all else be sure to test drive your headlines and track your results. If a headline is working, don't change it. If it stops working try something else.

You have to ensure your ad is read, the first time and every time. Flag them down and keep them reading.

These suggestions can be tailored to your business, just add the therapy, service or benefit you offer and utilise these headlines specific to your business. They really do work.

Why not try writing some headlines for your services using the previous examples now?

Chapter 10

Creative Copywriting

In this chapter we will explore how to write the content for your advertising that motivates your readers and give them every reason to book with you. Writing great copy is a skill but unless you want to employ the services of a professional copywriter there is no time like the present to begin. Nobody knows your practice like you do, which makes you the most qualified person to write about your services.

How to write great copy

When people think about writing copy they usually feel that this is beyond their ability but if you just imagine how you would talk to a friend about what you offer, the conversation is considerably more relaxed. There is no reason to put on a new face when writing as it will only come across as being phony.

To begin, I encourage you to record yourself describing the benefits of what you do and then transcribe your conversation into your advertisement. Of course, you will probably need to edit along the way but you'll find the nature of the writing is more intimate and personalised. It is about you expressing what you are passionate about and it expresses something that is totally unique because it comes from you.

The 4-step secret formula to making your ad work every time

Making your ad work means you need to capture the reader's attention and keep it. By utilising the following four steps you will have the ingredients you need to make your ad work every time.

The winning formula is:

1. **Attention**
2. **Interest**
3. **Solution**
4. **Action**

In order to have your ad read in the first place you need to arrest the reader's attention. This is done through writing an attention grabbing headline.

The second stage of the winning formula to making your ad work every time is to create interest. Here you pose the problem that your reader is having and identity with their situation.

The third stage is quite simple, offer a solution to their problem.

The fourth and final stage is the call to action where you state the benefits of taking action on the solution.

This formula can apply to almost any advertising.

Here's an example:

Got an aching back? – **Attention**

Did you know that over 40% of adults suffer from unnecessary back pain every day?

– **Interest**

Discover the tried and tested secret to relieving back pain in minutes. – **Solution**

Find out how you too can benefit, visit: www.backtobalance.com – **Action**

In this example, we flagged down the reader's interest with an attention grabbing headline. Anyone with back pain will read this headline and be compelled to read on.

In the second stage we have identified that the reader is not alone, other people have back pain but we are offering the reader something exclusive. In the third stage we offer the solution to the reader's problem, we reveal the secret to relieving back pain in minutes.

In the fourth stage we ask them to take action by finding out more via the website address.

It's that simple. By using the Attention, Interest, Solution, Action (AISA) formula you will be able to create an appealing solution to the reader's problems where they will be compelled to contact you.

In Joe Vitale's book 'Hypnotic Writing' he offers an alternative three step formula which I also like. His winning formula is: **Promise, Proof, Price.**

In Joe Vitale's example he uses **Promise** in the form of an attention grabbing headline, which offers something of interest to his reader.

The second stage is **Proof**. Here proof takes the form of a guarantee, testimonials, scientific studies or anything else which help convince the reader of the promise.

The third stage is **Price**. This is the buy now or call to action. In order to do this, it has to be an offer which cannot be refused, preferably with a limited time schedule.

For example: *'Book your first consultation before (insert date) and we'll give you a 50% discount, plus mention this ad to receive a free gift valued at $39.95! Hurry! Call 1800 234 555'.*

As you can see the formula is quite similar. Why not take a moment to write your own ad which utilises this formula. Do it now!

The length of your copy

Most people don't have the money to pay for large ads and as you have probably already discovered, the bigger the ad, the more you pay. However, it is not necessary to pay for large scale advertising in order to tell your story.

All you need to do is to lead readers to your website or email you for a free report or free newsletter. Don't be afraid of writing long copy. Tell a story and illustrate all of the benefits. Make it personal, relevant and compelling.

Generally, the higher the cost of your product or service, the longer the copy needs to be to sell the item. If you want someone to buy a $10,000 detoxification machine you'll need to write very long copy to convince your customer. However, if you are selling a half price treatment, your copy need not be so long.

The rule is: *'The more it costs, the more convincing you'll need to be'.*

Other tips for compelling copy

The following tips for compelling copywriting work wonderfully. If you have a story to tell, tell it by utilising some of these proven techniques.

Use emotional appeal

It is said that almost all of our buying decisions (in the end) are made based on emotions. Using emotional appeal is an excellent way to get inside your customer's head. When writing the copy for your advertisement it should appeal to the customer on an emotional level. If you can identify with their problems and strike an emotional chord you will retain their interest and they will want to find out more.

Use relevant quotes

Use relevant quotes in your writing. There may be a special quote from a famous person, healer, or mystic. Using quotes can inspire your reader and bolster your benefits at the same time.

Use analogies

Another useful technique is to draw analogies.
For example: *"Our treatment includes a soothing feather-light touch*

combining aromatherapy to drench your senses and lull you into a deeply relaxing state of being". Utilising words which create images and feelings can be a powerful way to capture the reader's imagination and produce a positive emotional response to your advertisement.

Ask questions

Have you ever noticed that when you read a question you have a response to that question already in your mind? Using a question in your advertising is an excellent way to establish a rapport with your reader. Simply ask a question related to your product or service and give an answer. For example, if you are an energy healer you could ask the question: *"Are you tired and lacking energy?"*. Once you ask the question you can then follow up with a subheading which offers the answer. Are you getting the idea?

Use repetition

Using repetition is also an excellent technique and a way of driving home your message. If you are writing very long copy your call to action can occur throughout the text. This way you give your reader every opportunity to act, rather than having to read all the way to the bottom of your message. If you have written your copy well you may find that the person will only read one quarter of the way down the page before they want to place an order. If you do not give them the opportunity along the way, you may lose them instead.

Use testimonials

Always use credible testimonials throughout your copy. Testimonials should be from customers who have utilised your services or products in the past. Testimonials instill confidence. A good amount is three or four. Testimonials add tremendous credibility to your offer.

Use boxes

> **Have you noticed
> that when something is written
> in a box, it suddenly becomes
> more appealing?**

Putting text inside a box is an excellent way to draw attention to an important piece of information and is also visually arresting. Putting a box around a special offer is an excellent way to draw attention to it, especially if you have a lot of copy.

Use a 'P.S.'

Another way to finish a long copy advertisement is to finish with a P.S. (post script), just in the same way that you would add a finishing note to a letter.

I don't know why it is but people just can't help but read a P.S. There is something very compelling about them.

Adding a 'P.S.' gives you the opportunity to remind your reader about your special offer or a final call to action which is time sensitive. I've also used P.P.S. with great effect, outlining a second special offer to follow up the first.

For example:

P.S. If you visit our website in the next 24 hours, you will receive an additional 20% off your next consultation.

P.P.S. Book a treatment before 5pm today and you will also receive an additional 10% off. That's a massive 30% off, but you must act before 5pm today!

Chapter 11

The Lifetime Value of your Clients

In this chapter I will explain how important repeat business is and how you can generate it by following some simple principles which will give you positive cash flow for years to come.

Many people underestimate the lifetime value of their clients and once they have received one booking, they are forever striving to obtain new clients. According to Fortune Magazine it costs five times as much to generate a new customer than it is to resell to an existing customer. Other sources have put the figure much higher to convert new business.

Your existing customer base is really a gold mine for your business. The problem is that most businesses fail to utilise their existing customers to resell. Your existing customers are the most pre-disposed to buy again from you because they already know what you offer.

Because your customer has had a previous experience and hopefully a positive one they know you will be able to provide a similar positive experience the next time they receive your treatment. In this way the element of risk is removed. This is why it is so important to offer exceptional service so when you contact your existing clients they will be happy to hear from you.

Once you have secured a new client and have given them a treatment, you really should bend over backwards to keep them happy. The reason for this is simple; if they are happy they will use your service not only again but several times and may tell many of their friends, who will also use your services in the future.

When you think about it, one treatment can translate into

dozens, just by providing excellent customer service and offering incentives to return or tell their friends. No other form of advertising works better than word of mouth and to not utilise this golden opportunity with your existing clients will lose you a great deal of on-going business.

In summary, the reasons an existing client is so valuable include:

1. **Already converted.** Meaning they are sold on the benefits of what you can offer, through direct experience.
2. **Repeat business.** They will bring in repeat business (provided they are happy with your sessions) by re-booking treatments in the future.
3. **Will tell their friends.** The most important of all three. If your treatments shine, they will invariably refer you to their friends and family members.

Following on from the third point is to give your clients an incentive to share. For example, you might offer them a 10% discount off their next treatment for every time they directly refer you a new client. Tell them to tell their friends to say: *"(Your client's name) was the one who told me about your treatments"*.

Alternatively, offer your client a free gift in the post and thank them for referring new people to you. They will not only be surprised to receive a formal thank you, they will also genuinely feel appreciated and this will invariably secure more appointments as well as on-going referrals in the future.

The real value of your customers

The fact of the matter is that your loyal customers want to buy from you again and again.

If we look at the lifetime value of a client it is easy to see why it is so important to offer exceptional customer service. To illustrate an example, let's say you charge $50 per treatment. If you give your client no opportunity to book again, at the end of the day all you have is $50. On the other hand, if you create opportunities where your client will book again and again, the lifetime value of your client can extend into the thousands.

Let us assume the same person comes back to you for regular treatments because you have offered them a special such as 'book five treatments for the price of four'. In this case, our client has turned into a $200 client every five weeks.

Let's take this a step further, let's say through your continued promotional efforts that your client comes every week taking advantage of the same offer for 12 months. For the sake of easy calculations, let's say that this is $200 per month for 12 months. In this case, your $50 client turns into a $2,400 client per year.

Now let us say you also sell some related products to the same client which they buy every week for $30, less your wholesale purchase price of $15, leaving you a $15 profit. $15 x 4 weeks is: $60 per month. Times this by 12 months = $720 a year. Add this to our total and the $50 client turns into a $3,120 client.

Now what if your client told five friends about you and they did the same thing? Your $50 client would now have made you $15,600.

It is interesting, isn't it?

Ah, but I hear you say, "It doesn't happen this way, not all five clients will do the same" and of course I agree with you, but what if only two did? What if those two clients, told three clients each, who told their friends who became clients? Can you see the potential?

The point is not that we see our clients only as numbers and income. The point I am trying to impress upon you is to give you some perspective on the scope of possibilities that come by utilising the right strategies as well as offering excellent treatments and customer service.

The reality is that you never know just how far one client can take your business so it is essential to be excellent at what you do and deliver this every time to every client.

You are only as good as your last treatment in the eyes of your client so remember this and do not slide into laziness or complacency with long term clients.

How to rekindle previous clients

The following suggestions are some additional ways which will help you rekindle the smoldering ambers of yesterday's clients.

Keep in touch every 90 days

Have you ever wondered why advertisers promote their product or service not once but several times? Keeping your service in front of your existing clients at least every 90 days reminds them that you still exist and that they should consider your services in the future. This can be easily achieved in one of the following ways.

Special offers

It cannot be stressed enough the importance of offering your existing clients a regular mail-out with an enticing special offer that is too good to ignore. By putting your name in front of your clients you become memorable and entice them to use your services again and again.

If you have a large client base you may consider a regular e-newsletter which they can subscribe and importantly unsubscribe to. This will save you time and money when it comes to stuffing envelopes and the costs of postage. With opted in customers online, renewed business is just one email away.

Preferred client club and VIP membership

Another way to encourage old clients is to offer them free VIP membership. As a part of this preferred clients' club they could be entitled to a free gift such as a 'two for one' offer every 90 days. VIP membership will also make your client feel like they are a very important person. You might even go to the trouble of making a laminated VIP preferred customer membership card or present them with a certificate of membership with their name printed on it. This can be sent to them as an attached file in PDF format or printed and posted at a small cost to your business.

The thing to remember is that we are in the business of building customer relationships so do what you can to make them feel special.

Send a postcard

Sending a postcard is another great way to stay in touch but it should relate to your business. Remember to personalize the message (hand written is preferable) and add a special offer on the back of the postcard which has a clear call to action or expiry date.

Sponsor an event

Sponsoring an event is another way to network your business plus offer something special to your existing clients. You may wish to sponsor an industry related information evening or combine sponsorship with a natural therapy college's open day. As a sponsor you can invite your existing customers for free or arrange a discount on related health products which may be of interest to them.

Happy birthday!

As part of your first consultation, request your new client's date of birth. This can be easily achieved when they fill out their client information form. Once you have obtained the client's birth date you can send them a special birthday notice each year. This may take the form of a genuine birthday gift or if they have not made a booking in months you might offer them a special which will entice them to repurchase from you.

Acknowledging birthdays is an excellent method to build

client relationships and to generate new business as a result. Again be sure to personalise birthday cards in your hand writing.

Anniversaries and special calendar dates

Anniversaries are another excellent way to bring in new business. It could be the anniversary date of their first treatment with you. Alternatively you can reward your customers with a free gift on their 20th treatment.

You can use other special calendar dates such as: Christmas; New Year; Chinese New Year; End of Financial Year; Valentine's Day; Mothers Day; Fathers Day; Halloween, or any other date you can think of. Be sure to tie in a great deal and make it interesting and unique to grab your client's interest.

We miss you!!!

Another excellent way to rekindle previous clients is to send them a 'we miss you' card or email. You may wish to write a letter something along the following lines:

Dear (person's name),

This letter is a little note to say that 'we miss you'. As a preferred client we wanted to bring to your attention a fabulous special offer. Because we value your business we would like to offer you 50% off your next treatment. Just mention this letter and make a booking before: (insert expiry date).

As an added bonus, if you tell a friend about our 50% off deal, we'll extend the same discount to them and give you a free gift pack valued at $30.00, just for sharing our great deal.

In order to receive your $30.00 free gift pack, make sure you ask your friend to mention that it was you who told them about our special offer and we will cheerfully post your gift within 14 days.

We sincerely hope to hear from you soon and look forward to offering you the best service and treatment you truly deserve.

To make your booking now and to secure your $30.00 free gift pack plus 50% off, e-mail us at (insert your email address).

Kind regards, (insert your name).

I recently sent a letter just like this one to my dormant clients and was amazed just how many responses I received within hours of sending it.

Exceptional customer service

If you want to maintain the life-time value of your client you need to offer not just customer service, but *exceptional* customer service. This means to exceed your customer's expectations, not just meet them.

When speaking with your clients over the phone, be friendly and polite and do your best to deliver the best possible service you can. When returning calls do your utmost to return them the same day, if not within the same hour the call was made.

If you are going to post your enquirer some information, over deliver on your promises. Make certain that they receive the information a day before they expect it. Remember, that when you get what you want, faster than you expect, it leaves you pleasantly surprised and satisfied with the service being offered.

When it comes to email, send the information as you are speaking to the client over the phone or as soon as you hang up. The customer has sought you out over your competition so don't disappoint them with late replies and slow deliveries.

When I receive enquiries I often email as I chat. Then I ask them to click 'send and receive' and hey presto! There is the email they require sitting in their inbox. This really makes a good impression.

When your client arrives for their treatment, offer them a drink (preferably water) and engage in some small chat*, asking them how they are or what they have been doing.

This not only keeps things on an intimate level it also sends a clear message to your client that you are interested in them as a person, not just as a client.

{One word of caution here is not to allow the chat time to go on for too long, as this will cut into your session time and the amount of time they have for their treatment.}

The power of thank you

Remember what your mother told you about please and thank you? Manners are important and by saying thanks at the end of your treatment, you really honour the person. Always thank your client at the end of the treatment for they are doing you a service just by being there. They offer you a valuable chance to refine and practice your abilities, plus they are also paying you for that opportunity. Saying thank you makes your client feel valued and respected.

Another thing you might consider on occasion is to offer your existing clients a thank you card in the mail or an e-card over the internet following the session. Again, this need not be a big deal it is just a little note to say thank you for their patronage.

The same applies when sending email. Remember to be courteous in all your correspondence and say thank you where possible. Be genuine as this really comes through even though it is email.

Remember your client's name

Another important point to make is that of remembering your client's name. Nothing is as de-valuing as forgetting a client's name or worse, calling them the wrong name. This includes making sure your client's name is spelled correctly when sending promotional materials. Whether these are letters or email correspondence, ensure you are correct in your spelling.

It is easy to relate to the power of remembering names. You need only think about how valued you feel when somebody remembers your name. The thing is we identify very strongly with our names. Names symbolise who we are and our name carries our innate vibration.

An excellent way to remember people's names is to associate their name with a word that rhymes with the name or associate a symbol or object with the name. It does take some practise to remember people's names, but you will be positively surprised how well they will respond to you when you do.

It is also advisable to take note of your last conversation with that person. Very often each client will have a client information sheet which you can update each visit.

Once the person has left make a few brief notes about the last treatment for your reference as well as what you discussed last time. They may have been going through some difficulty or were speaking about their pets or family members. Next time you see them you can pick up where you left off last time. Your client will feel pleased and reassured that you are taking an active interest in their life, (which you are) and this will engender a tremendously positive response.

The benefit of feedback

One of the most valuable things your clients can give you is constructive feedback. Never miss an opportunity to learn how you can improve the service you are offering.

One simple idea is to give your client a quick feedback sheet at the end of your session. Ask them if they wouldn't mind spending a minute to complete the tick box questionnaire.

The following is an example you may wish to use in conjunction with your treatments.

We value your comments and feedback.
Please take a moment to complete this feedback form.
Note: Your comments will be kept strictly confidential.

1. How would you rate your overall experience?
Poor / Average / Good / Very Good / Excellent

2. Did you feel this treatment represented value for money?
Yes / No

3. Did this treatment meet your expectations? **Yes / No**

4. What did you like most about this treatment?

_____

_____

5. What do you feel could be improved?

_____

_____

6. Other comments or suggestions?

_____

_____

7. Would you recommend our treatments to others? **Yes / No**

8. Would you like to offer a testimonial for use on our promotional materials? **Yes / No.** If Yes, please write your testimonial below:

_____

_____

_____

Thank you for taking the time to give your valued feedback!

Your name: _____

Contact number: _____

Email: _____

This feedback sheet is only a guide and you may wish to make changes to suit your treatments.

Once you have received several feedback sheets of this kind you will start to see where your business can be improved and make changes accordingly.

Another way to obtain feedback is to email this feedback form to your clients. If sending this in the post, be sure to include a postage paid self-addressed envelope so all they need to do is complete the form and post it back at no cost to them.

Following up on constructive criticism and being accountable

If you truly wish to make your services the best they can be then it makes sense to know what others think about what you do. When you obtain any feedback you should be more interested in what can be improved, than what is good about your service. Although it is nice to hear how much someone loved your session, it does not really help you to improve your service. What you really need to know is what is wrong with your service and then be able to take the necessary steps to improve it.

When you receive constructive criticism, don't take it personally. No one is perfect and we can always learn something new. If you have made an error, never try to worm your way out of it. Mistakes happen, details get lost, appointments are missed or your computer goes on the blink.

Things happen which are beyond your control. If something like this happens you need to let your customers know. Most will appreciate the honesty and will feel you care about them and the business relationship.

However, not to be accountable means you will lose the customer's respect and trust. They will feel betrayed and you may lose them as a customer for life.

Chapter 12

Networking your Business

Networking your business can open the door to new streams of business in ways you may never have expected. In this chapter I will illustrate a variety of networking methods to increase your clientele and expand your business.

Forming a strategic alliance

A great way to increase your business is to form a strategic alliance with other businesses. This is where you form an agreement between yourself and another practitioner or natural therapy college or natural therapy centre.

Once you have done this successfully there is no limit to the number of therapists you can extend this to. I myself have used this system well in the past and have successfully networked my practice with dozens of therapists.

The thing with strategic alliances is that you need to be sure it is reciprocal. The best way to test the water is to always ask who it was that referred you. Once you know the alliance is a two-way agreement in practise you have a 'win, win' scenario for all concerned.

Combined mail-out with other therapists

If you have done so already you'll already know that it can be really expensive doing mail outs to prospective clients, especially if the mailing list is extensive. Why not share the costs with fellow natural therapists and share expenses equally? This not only brings in a wider range of clients as you are sharing your database and their databases collectively, but you'll also be able to reduce your costs. It is a very good idea to ensure that you select the right client lists.

The important thing to remember is that each practitioner should have an equal advertising presence in the mail-out with equal opportunity to receive calls from the advertising. Each therapists phone numbers and email addresses should be featured on the promotional materials.

Coming together with other natural therapists who share a common goal to provide their services to many people can do very well using this strategy. Why not give it a try with the fellow practitioners you know?

Combined advertising

The same also applies for combined advertising. If you are advertising in a magazine and realistically all you can afford is a small space advertisement, by getting together with other practitioners and sharing the costs of a full page advertisement you will find that your presence in the publication will be far greater plus you'll have more space to sell yourself.

I recently saw an advertisement like this for *Pranic Healing* in our local new age magazine. The advertisement was a full page and eight practitioners were advertised. Each practitioner was listed in a specific location. The advertisement also featured the photographs of the individual practitioners and their phone number and email addresses were also listed. There was a lot of space to describe the benefits of the healing modality, which helped to sell the therapy and practitioners equally.

Referral rewards program

Having a referral rewards program is where you encourage your existing clients to share your business with others, but with a difference. We have touched on previous incentives such as discounts off their next treatment, but the difference here is that you actually pay your clients to share your services with friends and family. For example, each time a new person refers a friend and that friend books and pays as a direct result, you reward them with a referral bonus of a nominated amount.

In my business, *The International Institute for Complementary Therapists* (IICT) we utilise a Referral Rewards Program with excellent results. Each time an existing member refers someone to us and they in turn become members we transfer $10.00 into their bank account.

In order to track referrals we ensure that all of our membership application forms (both online and in hard copy) feature a space for the new applicant to type in the name and membership number of the person who referred them. We also provide our members with tools to share our business with others. This includes an online referral form where members can email friends about the IICT as well as information fliers offering a space to list the members name and membership number.

Whenever one of our members has referred a new customer, we contact them through our online database that they have been listed as a referrer. When notifying the member that they have been referred we also request their bank account details in order to make the internet banking transfer. The more times they refer the more we transfer into their account.

Why on earth would we do this? Well, the logic is simple. Everyone wins. If one of our members actively refer new clients to us we pay them each time. Five referrals equals $50 into the member's online account. We are happy to pay for the referrals because each time a new member joins it is one less person we need to advertise for. Plus in most cases the lifetime value of the client is a clear consideration.

Take a look at the following link: www.iict.com.au /referrals.htm and you will see that all the person needs to do is fill in the e-mail addresses of fellow practitioners to benefit.

In addition to referral bonuses we also give our members a number of free gifts once they qualified a certain number of referrals. These free gifts include movie passes, shopping gift vouchers, and iPod MP3 players to reward their efforts.

For more on our referral rewards program, take a look at this link to our website: www.iict.com.au/rewards-program.htm. Here all of the benefits are outlined for active referrers.

This may be a feature you can add to your website and reap the rewards of your clients making your business grow. How might you create a similar system which works for your business?

Expanding your client base

In order to reach a wider audience it is important to think outside the scope of what is considered normal forms of advertising. There are many places where your natural therapy can be of benefit and the following are some additional suggestions where you can not only source new clients but where you can extend your practice to the wider community.

Schools, universities and colleges

Why not contact your local school or university? You could offer treatments to *'stressed out'* exam students or to teachers who need time out from *stressed out* students. Many schools and universities have notice boards and these are ideal locations to advertise your services. Today many younger people have a deep interest in alternative therapies and you have a real opportunity to obtain new clients by advertising in this largely untapped market.

Beauty therapists, day spas, and health retreats

Beauty therapy centres, day spas and health retreats offer massage as well as many other forms of relaxation therapy. Why not offer your services as a practitioner? You may find that you will be able to gain a part-time position giving treatments and the benefit is that the centre will arrange your bookings and will have a suitable room for giving your sessions. Although you will not be paid at your usual rate, you will benefit from a regular clientele and this can often translate into private bookings. You may also be able to advertise in their monthly newsletter to expand your business.

Sports and recreation centres

Another largely untapped market is your local sports and recreation centre. Here your treatments can be advertised as assisting with the treatment of sports injury and increasing performance.

The fact is that there is a wealth of opportunities to share your services with the wider community. All you need to do is expand your thinking and pursue these possibilities to see which doors open.

Chapter 13

How to Grow your Business for Free

In this chapter I will share with you how to generate growth in your business without spending a cent. There are many possibilities to gain free publicity through a variety of means and the following examples provide some food for thought.

Writing articles

One excellent way to gain free exposure is through writing articles about your practice and having these published through local newspapers, new-age or holistic magazines and internet websites. Most magazines and newspapers are always looking for a feature article about a diverse array of subjects on a regular basis.

Writing an article on your area of expertise can boost your public profile as well as increasing public awareness of your profession. You can be a part of this by putting your fingers to work on the keyboard and getting your message out to the masses. You will be amazed at how a simple article will bring in a torrent of new clients from all walks of life.

To give you an example, one article I had published resulted in over 100 enquiries over the course of one week. This produced a stream of new clients and only cost me a small amount of my time to write the article. I still received calls from this article, months later.

Offering public talks

Offering public talks about your modality is another great way to increase your clientele and public profile. Try your local community centre, bookshop, healing centre or new age shop. If you are offering a talk at one of these venues, often they will promote your talk free of charge and this alone promotes your services to the wider community.

The best way to get higher numbers is to offer to give the talk free of charge. You might also look into some small notices in the local paper to get the word out. If you are offering a free talk some papers may even offer a free advertisement mentioning you in the 'what's happening' section.

When preparing your talk, be sure that you practice what you wish to say beforehand. Preparation is the key to giving a successful presentation. You may also consider reading some books on public speaking or do a short course on the subject to fine tune your presentation skills.

One way to structure a talk is to include some of the following points:

- An introduction of yourself and how you started in your modality
- Your background, qualifications and experience in your modality
- An overview of what you will be talking about
- The origins and history of your modality
- How a treatment is given
- The benefits of your treatments
- Give a short demonstration of the treatment or product (on a member of the audience)
- Offer a summary of what you have talked about
- Finish with question and answer time
- Give out your contact details and a special offer for your services

Once you have given your talk, you can also offer attendees further information by mail or email, as well as calling them for feedback with regards to your talk a few days later. In order to achieve this, be sure to have a contact list available before and after the talk. Also mention to the attendees that that they can fill in their details for more information or join your free newsletter.

Putting on a fundraising event

Another way to increase public awareness about you and your practice is to put on a fund raising event or raffle in conjunction with a non-profit charitable organisation. This could be a charitable ball or a raffle which includes your services as a prize.

Riding on the back of other well known charities is a great way to give your practice an enormous boost because many have the resources, funding, and especially extensive databases where you will be mentioned.

'Tryvertising'

This following strategy will work wonders in your practice and it has been used successfully by many practitioners for decades. It is a little bit like advertising, except you get to 'try before you buy'.

It's a simple idea that costs you little in advertising and is an excellent way to generate new clients and retain them. As we have discussed, it can be very difficult to obtain new clients so one way to generate them is by giving them a free treatment or consultation.

Think about it, if you are any good at what you do, the likelihood is that they will book with you again. As they are not required to pay any money the only thing that they are risking is their time. This strategy works very well provided you implement a follow-up strategy.

There is the possibility that some people will take advantage of the free treatment and not return but most people are genuinely interested and this can be the very thing that gives them permission to try your therapy for the first time.

Instead of looking at the time we lose by giving away free treatments, we need to look at the benefits and what we will receive. The end result is new clients who will pay again and again.

There are several ways to promote *Tryvertising*. A simple way is to upgrade the treatment. For example, your first half hour is free and then they are given the opportunity to upgrade their treatment session to a full hour for a reduced fee.

For example, if you are at naturopath, your first consultation could be free and during this consultation time you have an opportunity to show your new client the benefits and where they could go from there.

You could also offer supplements that will support their health and well-being and make additional income selling products.

Chapter 14

Alternative Ways to Market your Business

In this chapter I will share with you some additional ways to market your natural therapy business without needing to wear a chicken costume to stand out.

Fake cheque

A great way to market your business in conjunction with a special offer is to create a fake cheque. The important thing to note here is that the cheque is a fake and not a direct copy from an existing bank. A cheque addressed to the recipient with a dollar amount is instantly attention grabbing.

The reason for this is that our minds instantly associate cheques with money, so they are less likely to be ignored. I have used fake cheques for years and I have always found them to be an excellent visual way to attract new clients to a special offer.

A word of warning, it is especially important to state on your cheque that it is not redeemable through any bank. It may seem obvious but if you are going to create a fake cheque you need to ensure that you are not going to be up for fraud as a result. Also be aware not to breach copyright of banks' logos. There can be very serious penalties for such breaches of copyright and banks would not take kindly to such infringements being made.

On the fake cheque, place a dollar amount which might be for example - $100.00.

In this case the cheque is payable to the recipient stating your special offer which might read: *"Register for a treatment package before (state expiry date) and receive $100.00 of additional pamper treatments for free"*.

Get your business into the Guinness Book of World Records

It may seem like a crazy idea but if you can achieve a new world record the publicity could be tremendous. Perhaps you could do a 24-hour treatment or try and treat as many people as possible in one hour. The possibilities are only limited to your imagination.

If you do manage to get your business into the Guinness Book of World Records in relation to your natural therapy practice you can utilise this achievement in your future advertising. It is also an excellent way to attract media attention, which translates into free publicity.

If you are planning on setting a new record be sure to attract the media and send out a press release to all the major newspapers and local television stations. Even if you don't get into the Guinness Book of World Records your attempt would certainly be newsworthy. You can start your journey at: www.guinnessworldrecords.com

Cater to parents

Another largely untapped market is to cater your natural therapy practice for parents with babies or children. You might offer natural therapy treatments at your local child care centre or health club which has a crèche. While the children are playing the parents can enjoy a natural therapy treatment. This way you can advertise through your local health club or child-care centre and tap into a whole new market.

There are so many opportunities out there and all you need to do is start exploring.

One shiatsu practitioner I know offers shiatsu for pregnant women. She has a simple flyer which she has inserted into the hospitals' pregnancy package at the birthing centre. Every new pregnant mum-to-be receives a brochure offering an introductory shiatsu treatment.

Some other untapped markets include: the elderly; child-care centres; health clubs; charities; on-site office treatments; and festivals.

I suggest you take a look around at what is going on in your community and think of some of the new ways that you can offer your natural therapy treatment to a wider market. You will receive some rejections but with perseverance you certainly will receive some positive responses as well.

Create a promotional CD

Making a promotional CD is not necessarily an expensive exercise. One low cost option is to record a CD where you are interviewed about the benefits of your natural therapy practice by a friend or colleague. During the interview you can give answers to the questions which present the benefits of what you offer.

Alternatively, your CD may be a free report where you explain the benefits about what you offer. In a similar way to presenting a talk about your natural therapy business, you can type the script then read it into a recorder and burn this to CD's. These days it's very easy to produce a low-budget CD from your personal computer.

You can also use an MP3 player and save the recording as a file downloaded to your computer. As your enquiries come in all you have to do is burn copies of your free report and send these out with your promotional materials. It is also easy to print professional looking labels from most printers. When you purchase labels for CD's there is often software which accompanies the labels. From under two dollars you can produce a free CD giveaway.

Once produced, you can then advertise this CD as a free report valued at $37.00. The value you place on your CD is entirely up to you.

Alternatively, if you want to professionally produce 100 or

more CD's the price can be reduced but minimum orders usually apply. A quick search on Google.com will provide several options of companies who can produce your promotional CD at a reasonable cost.

Write a book

It sounds like a big project to write a book and to be honest it does take time. However, if you can hold a conversation about the benefits of your natural therapy and have some sound expertise and experience, you have what it takes to become an author. There are some considerable benefits to writing a book.

When you write a book you instantly move from being a natural therapy practitioner to someone who has credibility. In the eyes of the public and your peers you become an authority on your subject and this can be used to your advantage. As an author you can advertise this on your promotional materials and sell your book on the internet.

To begin only two things stand in your way. The first is writing the book and the second is having your book published. As it may not be easy to have your book published, so many people now choose to go down the road of self-publishing either in print or as an e book.

Publishing an e book is the most cost effective way as it is simply an electronic format that can be downloaded from your website or emailed as a PDF. If you self-publish in print then the costs are far higher. Prices usually start from several hundred dollars depending upon the print run to thousands. If you do self-publish, you may find it takes some time to sell or even give away 500 to 1000 copies. I recommend the e-book approach as being the best solution. An easy way to write your book is to utilise voice recognition software through your personal computer. Most people cannot type at the speed of light so a good alternative is to utilise a program such as *Dragon Naturally Speaking* – visit: www.nuance.com. The first draft of this book was dictated using the same software.

Here you can dictate your book in real time as the words appear on your computer screen. Voice recognition software has come a long way in recent years and you can speak at regular talking speed with quite good accuracy using such programs. There will always be a certain amount of editing to complete your manuscript. I always recommend giving your completed manuscript to a number of people who can give you some honest feedback. They may also be able to assist you with editing the book to ensure that your book is something of quality.

Bear in mind that your book does not need to be hundreds of pages long. The number of pages you should aim for is somewhere between 100 to 120 pages long or 30,000 to 40,000 words. The internet can provide some excellent resources on writing, marketing and publishing your book so before you embark upon this prestigious and somewhat frustrating journey, I suggest you do your research well but most importantly – begin.

Offer a giveaway

Magazines love free giveaways. If you have written an e-book or produced a CD you have a quality product with a real value. This is perhaps one of the best free advertising tools at your disposal. Contact all of the alternative therapy magazines and newspapers and offer your book or CD as a free giveaway.

You may be able to exchange the giveaway for an article or book or CD review. If the magazine profiles your product (which ultimately sells you and your business) you have landed some free advertising.

Some ways to pitch your free giveaway include:

- a free copy with every 12 month subscription
- a free copy as part of a competition
- a free copy for the best letter to the editor.

Whichever way the magazine wants to give your product away is of no concern of your's, the fact of the matter is you will have gained valuable free publicity and advertising plus a stream of new clients as a direct result.

Chapter 15

Expanding your Business

This chapter will take your business to the next level, from sole operator to business owner. I will explain how best to support and reward your staff, including training and incentives as well as presenting numerous income streams for your business.

After utilising a great many recommendations from this book your business will be booming. The only problem being is that there is only one of you and with so many new clients coming your way you need help. Because of all the hours you are doing you probably feel like you need a holiday too.

The problem that most business owners encounter is that they are experts at what they do. This means that nobody else can do what they do. If nobody can replace them this also means that they are effectively 'married' to their business.

Many practitioners who become very successful end up working very long hours, sometimes seven days a week with little time for family or a social life.

The solution is to take on staff who are trained in such a manner to deliver the same level of quality service as you offer and thereby lighten your workload. With additional staff working in your business you then have time to work on your business not just in it.

This does not mean that you no longer give treatments, but you'll have a choice to take a break, have a holiday and do less hours as and when it suits you. The added benefit of taking on staff is that you will be making more. Sure you have to pay your staff but more sessions equates to more profits, provided you do it the right way.

So how do we train our staff to give the quality treatments our existing clients have come to love? We achieve this by training our staff with a systems operations manual*.

A systems operations manual is a step-by-step guide of how your business is run. If your staff have a guide to follow which ensures every level of service is conducted the way you wish it to be, from picking up the phone and answering calls to giving a treatment and everything in between, you can be assured you will be able to replicate yourself and reap the rewards accordingly.

Working on your business is looking into how to consistently offer a more refined service as well as continually striving to find new ways to improve and market your business. With more time to attract new clients and look after your existing clients your turnover can increase as well as your profits, even though you are paying staff wages.

*See: www.e-myth.com

Taking on staff

When you are considering taking on staff, you need to determine just how many you will need. If you are taking this step for the first time I recommend you take on not one but two staff members at the same time. This way if one leaves or is sick you have a back up practitioner who can fill in. It is called spreading your risk.

You will also need to define what your staff will be expected to do as well as determining how you will operate your business from this new paradigm.

The first thing you need to do is to ensure that staff has an appropriate level of training so that they can perform and offer a similar level of service and quality. When advertising the positions available you will need to be clear from the outset how much you will be willing to pay your staff, whether it is on a per treatment basis or hourly wage. You will also need to determine the tasks your staff will be expected to perform. Will they be expected to open the clinic, do the banking and buying of clinic supplies, or will they just conduct treatments and nothing more?

When making your selection of a new staff member it is important to take your time in the selection process and this includes interviewing your applicant and doing a full background check.

You may also wish to have a checklist or 'wish list' of the types of qualifications you require as well as determining whether your applicant has the necessary people skills.

Your checklist may include:

- Skills – what level of skills are necessary for the position. This includes not only the qualifications but being able to demonstrate an appropriate level of proficiency in conducting a treatment or consultation. One way to check the applicant skill level is to have them facilitate a treatment on you as if you were a client.

- History – what prior experience have they had in the natural therapy industry and can they supply any references to support this. Be sure to review their resume and be aware that most resumes are impressive but can be somewhat fictional.

- References – does the applicant have any references?

- Presentation – how do they present themselves when interviewed? Do they arrive late and is their personal appearance clean and tidy? You will need to observe them carefully and trust your gut feeling.

- Attitude – does this person have a 'can do' attitude and do they have a passion for this work? It is also important to know your staffs' hobbies and interests outside the work environment as well as any health or relationship issues which may affect their overall performance.

- Pressure – how do they perform under pressure or when difficult situations arise? How do they resolve issues with client complaints and do you have systems in place for resolving such issues if and when they arise?

If your applicant does not meet these base standards my advice is do not hire them. If you begin by making exceptions from the beginning there is no telling how many problems will develop in the future.

At the same time you cannot expect your staff to know everything from the start. As with any new business there will always be a certain amount of on-the-job training and the more you can be clear about the tasks required (having written these down in a concise manner in your systems operations manual), the more likely you'll avoid problems with your employees in the future.

Rewarding your staff

When it comes to paying your staff you want to ensure that they are appropriately rewarded for their efforts. Offering special staff incentives is an excellent way to acknowledge their efforts. If your staff enjoy their work and feel acknowledged and valued they will be happy to work with you for years to come.

This is why it is vital to recruit staff who have the right mind set to begin with. If they have a passion for their natural therapy and feel they are offering a genuine service to their clients they will continue to work for you, even without a high wage, so long as you offer the right incentives and regularly reward their loyalty.

You can do your part to help your staff help your business by offering them inspiration and by being a living example of how you want your business to be. You want to paint a picture in their minds that is one of excellent customer service and attention to detail.

This is imparted through your training and reviewed on a regular basis. This is especially important during the first few months as they begin to find their way working in your business.

The other ways you can support your staff is by treating them like shareholders and not your employees. What do I mean by this?

The view should be that of a team mentality where you welcome their thoughts and ideas of how the business can be run better. This way they will feel like a team player and will have more energy for the business as a whole.

Feedback from your staff

Just as it is important to give feedback to your staff on their performance and to gently mentor changes where needed, it is equally important to receive feedback from your staff. This is something that you should do on a semi-regular basis.

Asking your staff for feedback on how your business is being conducted as well as reviewing how the business is running promotes shareholder mentality and makes your staff feel they are a valuable asset to the business.

Welcome feedback on what areas need improving and if you feel these are appropriate suggestions implement them and review the progress on a regular basis. It is very easy to become complacent in your business when all is going well. However, complacency breeds all kinds of problems in a business which appears to be coasting along. Real growth comes from diligent attention to all areas of your business. Remember to always keep your finger on the pulse to keep offering exceptional customer service.

Review your staff progress every three months

You need to review your staffs' needs and performance at least every three months, ideally sooner. This need not be a grueling interrogation, rather it is a time to touch base with how they are going and being open to hearing their suggestions. Although you are officially the boss you should approach things as a team, as your staff are the life blood of your business.

Always treat them like this and you'll grow a positive empire which benefits all concerned. In addition to three-monthly reviews, (depending upon the number of staff) you may choose to review progress monthly or even weekly. This is something you will need to determine according to the nature of your business.

Moving from practitioner to business owner

There may come a time when you move from being a practitioner working in your business to stepping aside entirely. This means that you are no longer facilitating treatments and move to a managerial position, or even appointing a manager of your business.

Moving from practitioner to business owner may not be everybody's wish as many people enjoy contact with their clients on a one-to-one basis. The thing is you can have your cake and eat it. Being a business owner means you can choose when you give treatments and when you work. How much you do becomes your choice.

If you wish to write yourself out of the picture entirely and free up your time to pursue other projects then you'll need some clear systems in place to do so. If this is your goal then I recommend you take a look at two books in particular.

These are:

- The 4 Hour Work Week by Tim Ferriss. See: www.fourhourworkweek.com

- The Invisible Entrepreneur by Louise Woodbury and William De Ora.

See: www.take3months.com

Additional tips for business owners

In addition to the suggestions I have outlined in this chapter the following are some helpful tips for business owners that will keep your business in check and will help it stay healthy for years to come.

Have a good accountant

Having a good accountant is a must for running any business. By good I mean an accountant who is pro-active in finding ways to legally minimise your tax, as well as giving you the best returns and advice on how you can plan ahead for the future of your business. Sadly, most people address the books of the business as a last measure and deal with the tax problem at the end of each financial year.

This means that you will not have the necessary opportunities to reduce your tax legally by implementing structures such as forming a company or family trust which not only helps to protect your assets from litigation, they also offer excellent ways to reduce the amount of tax you have to pay.

I have mentioned the word 'legal' in that there are many legal ways to reduce tax without breaking any laws or placing yourself or your business at risk. My advice is to talk to your accountant about the future of your business and its projected returns and establish the necessary systems in advance.

I review my business plan every three months and track my expenses as well as profits monthly. Have your fingers on the pulse with your business through regular reviews and planning. Be sure to talk to your accountant and see what they can do for your business by thinking ahead.

Your intellectual property, trademarks and copyright

In the case where you have established a logo or trademark for your business or have materials such as manuals, promotional materials, systems operations manual and the like, you may wish to consider establishing copyright in order to protect your intellectual property.

It has been my experience that if you write a good brochure or produce a great logo that some unsavory people out there will think: 'Wow, that looks great, I'll use that for my business'.

Establishing copyright for your materials acts as a red flag for potential plagiarism or copy-cat practitioners grabbing your good ideas and creating materials for their benefit without compensating your talents.

In the case where you have written a manual, such as one for a workshop or course, as well as your advertising brochure and website content, one simple way to ensure that you created the materials when you did is to make copies and post these to yourself registered by mail or email. That way, if in the future you see your advertisement appear word for word (as I have experienced) without your written consent you will have proof of the original work prior to the appearance of copied material.

Because the material is officially post dated at the postal office, this is one legal way to ensure copyright is retained. One word of advice, however, is don't open your letter to yourself as this voids the seal of the date of publication. Another way is to email copies of your work to yourself prior to publication. This will also feature a date when sent to your inbox.

As the laws which govern copyright and trademarks vary as well as change from time to time, check with your local small business or ministry of fair trading office to see what options are available in your country.

Retain a good credit rating

In short, make sure you pay your bills on time. This includes the rent for your premises, your telephone bills and any other bills, especially with the banks. Your credit rating follows you throughout life. If you have a dispute with a service provider and receive a bad credit rating, this rating will never leave you. If you pay your bills on time you will be in the good books with your service providers and in the future you will have an easier time when applying for a business, home or investment loan with any bank.

The idea is that once you have made all the money from implementing the suggestions presented in this book, you can invest your profits in property, shares or a new business venture. It is wise counsel to seek the right advice if you wish to invest your hard-earned cash in other ventures. Having investments besides your business helps to spread your risk should anything go wrong with you or your business in the future.

Maintaining industry relationships
It should now come as common sense to be on good terms with your clients but we should extend this to our fellow industry professionals, wholesalers, suppliers, and especially the editors of mind body spirit type publications.

By maintaining good relations with fellow industry professionals you can form strong alliances and benefit from cross referrals as well as help build a name for your business for the future. The last thing you want is enemies. If you have bad relationships with fellow practitioners and maintain a small minded, competitive attitude, your business will ultimately fail. Bad news whether it is directed at you or from you travels at high speed and even faster in smaller towns. Always do your best not to enter into gossip or give disparaging remarks about other people within your industry or your staff.

There is no telling where stories go and the outcomes can be destructive for your business relationships. Ultimately we should be in the mindset that supports growth and mutual tolerance for one another. There is nothing to be gained from an overly competitive attitude.

When it comes to wholesalers and suppliers, good relationships means you will get to hear about special deals and will have the opportunity for extended 60 to 90 day accounts. This helps to keep your cash flow positive, which means you'll get your products without paying for everything up-front.

Lastly, maintaining excellent relationships with magazine editors and staff mean you'll get more good advertising discounts, special offers and bonuses as well as the *holy grail* – free publicity in the form of articles, reviews and features. Treat editors like gold as they are a lasting resource for your business success.

Review your business plan every three months

Review your business plan every three months. This includes tracking your advertising and marketing to see what worked and what did not work. Look at different ways to re-think your business and see how you might improve things.

Constantly strive to think outside the box to improve your business. If you change nothing you become stagnant and your business will go rancid in no time.

As part of your overall business health check, address the following questions at least every three months, these are:

- How effective is my marketing plan?
- What are the results of my marketing plan – what is working and what needs changing?
- How many enquiries and bookings resulted from my advertising efforts?
- What are the future directions of my business?
- Have I updated my goal list?
- What new innovations can I implement to expand my horizons?

- Is there anything which needs updating in my operations manual?
- Have I contacted my existing clients in the last 90 days?
- Have I asked my existing customers for referrals?
- Are my promotions materials up to date and is there adequate supply?
- Are my accounts and paperwork up to date?
- Are my staff happy and what changes are necessary?

These are just some of the questions you should ask yourself on a regular basis.

Chapter 16

Setting Goals for your Business

In this chapter we will examine what underpins a successful business which is regularly setting goals. Having the mindset for success in your business, as well as having personal and spiritual goals, can fast track your business to greater heights and fulfill your personal dreams.

Okay, so you've made it this far and now have all *the Secrets of Spiritual Marketing*. The thing is that having the tools to effectively market and advertise your natural therapy business is one thing, but if you lack the mental and emotional mind-set to allow prosperity and success, you are limiting your maximum prosperity potential.

The journey to personal and spiritual wealth
The journey to personal and spiritual wealth cannot be found on the outside. You can read all the books, apply all the mythologies, attend all the workshops and you will certainly gain knowledge and tools but unless you address your underlying issues around 'lack' your full potential will never be realised. As many of us grew up, we had negative re-enforcements about prosperity and money pushed on us.

If you have issues around money you may wish to do some personal development in this area. These core beliefs can hold you back and just in the same way you can implement changes in your business and create programs for success so it is with your beliefs around money.

This book is not intended to present a detailed analysis of one's core beliefs around prosperity. There is a tremendous body of work already published on this subject.

If you have prosperity issues, I strongly encourage you to explore this with a trusted therapist in order to break the beliefs that hold you back. There are many talented practitioners who can assist you in healing and growing in this case which go well beyond my suggestions.

Setting goals

In my experience, setting goals is one of the best ways to track your business success and is an excellent motivator to getting things done. If your goals remain simply as ideas in your head this is usually where they stay. You have to take the goals out of your head and put them on paper or in a visible document on your desktop computer where they will be there reminding you to complete them.

When interviewing successful business people in nearly every instance one of the primary reasons they achieved success in their business was the attention to goal setting and the systematic approach to achieving these goals. Research shows that on average only as little as 14% of people establish goals for their lives and barely 3% have their goals clearly defined in writing.

Beyond setting the primary goals, you should also include goals which at the present time exceed your comprehension to achieve them. This is part of your grand vision. You need to have a grand vision because you never know you may one day just find yourself living those lofty heights. These grand vision goals have a surprising ability to sneak up on you but they usually take a few years to manifest.

Like anything in life, you need to get to work on your goals for them to manifest. It is not enough to write them down then go back to watching the television every night and doing nothing to achieve your goals. I call this *'meeting spirit half way'*. You need to be active and work towards your goals and step-by-step you will eventually arrive. All you need is desire, expectation and the personal will to achieve these goals. By taking baby steps you will achieve them one at a time.

Goal setting is like taking a long journey. First you need to make plans; do your research; obtain your travel insurance; buy your travel tickets; and, pack your items for travel. Then you need to get to the airport, board your plane, and arrive at your chosen destination. It is not realistic to think that all that happens instantaneously, you need to take the small steps, one by one, and finally you arrive.

Arriving at a successful business is much the same. You need to take the necessary steps and do the hard yards in order to arrive in a successful business that will support you and your family for the years to come. Just in the same way that a farmer does not realise the crop the same day he sows the field, so it is with achieving your goals.

I know these are a few too many analogies, but I am trying to make my point crystal clear: **You have to take action systematically to realise your goals.** No one will do it for you. It is up to you to make a path for yourself.

Writing a goal list

I personally write and re-write goals on a monthly basis. These are set out into monthly, yearly as well as grand vision goals. I usually set these out in point form and at the end of each month I take a look at my goal list and tick off which ones have been achieved. The ones that have not been achieved I transfer to the next goal list for the month to come.

By just doing this one thing you will be able to achieve remarkable results both in your business and personal life and join the 3% of people who have their goals clearly defined in writing.

The other important step is to set dates when your goals will be achieved. Here I recommend you set slightly unrealistic dates. For example, when I undertake to write a book my publisher sets a date when the manuscript is due. In most cases this is not up for negotiation as a number of people are relying on me to have my manuscript ready by the due date. This naturally adds some pressure which in fact is a good thing.

What happens is when we set time limits on our goals a funny thing happens – we end up achieving them sooner than we expected.

I strongly encourage you to set deadlines to all your goals. It does not matter if you do not meet all your deadlines as you can always re-set the dates and move them to the following month. If you do not set dates, it is like you are saying to the universe, *"here is my goal, anytime you want to present the outcome is fine with me"*.

If this is your attitude then that is okay but if you want to achieve the same thing in one month that takes one year, it is up to you to claim it as so.

The universe will deliver but you need to give it a delivery time and a delivery address, otherwise your outcome will remain somewhere out in space and never land in your life.

When writing your goals list include all of the baby step goals along the way. These are the small steps which will enable you to fulfill the grand vision you have for yourself.

In addition to my monthly goals, I also set daily goals. In this way I move from being my usual lazy self to being *Lawrence the accomplisher!*

Working step-by-step in this way really helps you to achieve what you want in your practice and your personal life as well. The thing is you need to be clear on what you want and then get busy on how you will achieve it.

Your online goal list

If you are not so much into words for goals, another option is to create a vision board. This is where you put your goals into symbols and images.

You can take a great deal of time cutting out images from

magazines or words from newspapers but a far faster way is to create a series of images, symbols and words by surfing the internet and placing these images into a designated *my pictures* goal document. This then becomes your online goal list.

Every time you have a new goal, add a symbol or image which relates to this goal and save it to your image folder. You can add anything which is meaningful to you and your business. Now set your image goal folder as your screen saver slide show.

As soon as you are idle at your computer for more than a few minutes, your goals will pop up as a slide show reminding you about your goals and this will motivate you to get back to achieving them.

You can also default your favourite inspirational piece of music to launch with the screen saver to add to the overall experience. Give it a go and you'll be surprised just how effective this really is.

In summary

Throughout this book I have shared with you many well guarded *Secrets of Spiritual Marketing*. You now have the tools to make a definitive difference to your natural therapy business and the lives your business can touch. All you need to do is implement these recommendations into your practice and see the growth unfold in and around you.

To finish I wish you well on your journey and may you carry with you *the Secrets of Spiritual Marketing* throughout your expansive natural therapy career.

Happy healing!

Lawrence Ellyard

Resources and recommended reading lists

If you are genuinely interested in furthering your spiritual knowledge about prosperity as well as accessing some excellent marketing, small business, and entrepreneurial guides then I highly recommend the following books:

- Rich Dad, Poor Dad – by Robert T. Kiyosaki
- The Cashflow Quadrant – by Robert T. Kiyosaki
- Think and Grow Rich – by Napoleon Hill
- The Dynamic Laws of Prosperity – by Catherine Ponder
- The Magic of Thinking Big – David J. Schwartz
- The Ultimate Marketing Toolkit – Paula Peters
- You were Born Rich – Bob Proctor
- Grow your Business in 90 Days – Wendy Evans
- The Invisible Entrepreneur – Louise Woodbury and William De Ora
- The 4 Hour Work Week – Timothy Ferriss
- E-Myth Mastery – Michael E. Gerber
- The E-Myth Revisited – Michael E. Gerber
- The Success Principles – Jack Canfield
- Permission Marketing – Seth Godin
- The Big Red Fez – Seth Godin
- How to grow your business without spending a single cent – Justin Hearld
- Prosperity on Purpose – Justin Hearld
- Hypnotic Writing – Joe Vitale
- The 7 Habits of Highly Effective People – Stephen R. Covey
- Small Business Marketing for Dummies – Barbara Findlay Schenck
- Marketing Tips for Complementary Therapists: 101 Tried and Tested Ways to Attract and Retain Clients – Steven A.

Harold

- Ultimate Small Business Marketing Guide – James Stephenson

Other books by Lawrence Ellyard

The Spirit of Water – O Books Publishing (UK)
Everyday Buddha – O Books Publishing (UK)
Reiki Meditations for Beginners – O Books Publishing (UK)
Reiki 200 Questions and Answers for Beginners – O Books
Publishing (UK)
The Ultimate Reiki Guide for Practitioners and Masters – O
Books Publishing (UK)
Reiki Healer – Lotus Press (USA)

Guided meditation CD's by Lawrence Ellyard

Reiki Samadhi – Japanese Reiki Meditations – Reiki Soundz
(Australia)
The Spirit of Water – Guided Meditations – Hado Publications
(Australia)

Author website information

For more about these titles, reviews and author appearances
visit Lawrence Ellyard's author site at:

www.lawrenceellyard.com

Professional affiliation for natural therapists

The International Institute for Complementary Therapists, of
whom the author is the founder and director, offers
membership and professional affiliation for over 550 natural
therapy modalities throughout Australia and New Zealand. You
can find out more information by visiting: www.iict.com.au

Other websites from Lawrence Ellyard

The International Institute for Reiki Training:
www.reikitraining.com.au

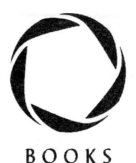

BOOKS

O is a symbol of the world, of oneness and unity. In different cultures it also means the "eye," symbolizing knowledge and insight. We aim to publish books that are accessible, constructive and that challenge accepted opinion, both that of academia and the "moral majority."

Our books are available in all good English language bookstores worldwide. If you don't see the book on the shelves ask the bookstore to order it for you, quoting the ISBN number and title. Alternatively you can order online (all major online retail sites carry our titles) or contact the distributor in the relevant country, listed on the copyright page.

See our website **www.o-books.net** for a full list of over 500 titles, growing by 100 a year.

And tune in to myspiritradio.com for our book review radio show, hosted by June-Elleni Laine, where you can listen to the authors discussing their books.

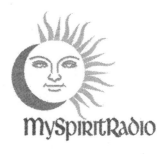